CHAIR YOGA FOR WEIGHT LOSS

FOR SENIORS OVER 60

Chair Yoga Mastery: 28 days of weight loss with low impact exercises for elderly men,women and beginners to increase strength, mobility and balance

By

DR.Ashley McGrane

Table of contents

<u>Introduction: Why Chair Yoga?</u>

Chair yoga is an accessible and beneficial form of yoga that offers numerous advantages, especially for those with limited mobility or who spend prolonged periods sitting. It provides a gentle way to improve flexibility, strength, and posture while reducing stress and promoting relaxation. Whether you're looking to incorporate gentle movement into your daily routine, alleviate tension from sitting at a desk, or simply enhance your overall well-being, chair yoga offers a convenient and effective solution.

Chair yoga is a modified form of traditional yoga that can be practiced while seated on a chair or using a chair for support. It incorporates gentle stretches, breathing exercises, and mindfulness techniques that can be easily adapted to accommodate various fitness levels and physical abilities.

Some key benefits of chair yoga include:

1. Improved Flexibility and Mobility: Chair yoga helps increase flexibility and range of motion by gently stretching and moving the body in a seated position. This is particularly beneficial for individuals with limited mobility or joint issues.

2. Enhanced Strength: Although chair yoga is gentle, it still engages muscles throughout the body, helping to improve strength, especially in the core, back, and legs.

3. Better Posture: Regular practice of chair yoga can help improve posture by strengthening the muscles that support the spine and encouraging proper alignment while sitting.

4. Stress Reduction: Chair yoga incorporates deep breathing and relaxation techniques that promote stress relief and relaxation. It can help calm the mind, reduce anxiety, and improve overall mental well-being.

5. Increased Energy and Vitality: By promoting better circulation and releasing tension, chair yoga can leave you feeling more energized and revitalized, even after a short practice session.

6. Accessibility: Chair yoga is suitable for people of all ages and fitness levels, including seniors, office workers, individuals with disabilities, and those recovering from injury or surgery. It can be easily modified to accommodate specific needs and limitations.

7. Convenience: One of the great advantages of chair yoga is its convenience. It can be practiced virtually anywhere – at home, in the office, or even while traveling – as long as you have access to a chair.

Overall, chair yoga offers a gentle yet effective way to improve physical and mental well-being, making it a valuable addition to any wellness routine. Whether you're looking to incorporate more movement into your day, manage stress, or simply take better care of your body, chair yoga provides a accessible and enjoyable option for all.

<u>Benefits of Chair Yoga for Seniors Over 60</u>

Chair yoga offers numerous benefits for seniors over 60, including:

1. Improved Flexibility: Chair yoga helps seniors increase flexibility by gently stretching muscles and joints, promoting mobility and range of motion.

2. Enhanced Strength: Through a series of seated poses and movements, chair yoga helps seniors build and maintain muscle strength, which is crucial for daily activities and balance.

3. Better Posture: Practicing chair yoga can help seniors develop better posture by strengthening core muscles and increasing awareness of body alignment while sitting.

4. Stress Reduction: Chair yoga incorporates breathing exercises and relaxation techniques that can help seniors manage stress, reduce anxiety, and promote a sense of calm and well-being.

5. Pain Relief: Seniors often experience joint pain and stiffness. Chair yoga can help alleviate these discomforts by gently stretching and releasing tension in targeted areas, such as the neck, shoulders, and back.

6. Improved Circulation: Chair yoga incorporates gentle movements and stretches that can improve blood circulation, which is important for overall cardiovascular health and preventing conditions like blood clots and varicose veins.

7. Enhanced Balance and Stability: Chair yoga includes poses and exercises that focus on balance and stability, helping seniors reduce the risk of falls and maintain independence in their daily activities.

8. Social Interaction: Participating in chair yoga classes provides seniors with opportunities for social interaction, reducing feelings of isolation and loneliness, and fostering a sense of community and belonging.

9. Accessible and Safe: Chair yoga is accessible to seniors of all fitness levels and physical abilities. It can be modified to accommodate individual needs and limitations, making it a safe and inclusive form of exercise.

10. Mind-Body Connection: Chair yoga emphasizes the connection between the mind and body, promoting mindfulness and self-awareness, which can contribute to overall mental and emotional well-being in seniors over 60.

11. Improved Breathing: Chair yoga incorporates breathing exercises (pranayama) that focus on deep, mindful breathing. This can help seniors improve lung function, increase oxygen intake, and promote relaxation.

12. Better Sleep Quality: Regular practice of chair yoga, particularly relaxation techniques and gentle stretches before bedtime, can help seniors improve sleep quality and manage insomnia or sleep disturbances commonly experienced with age.

13. Enhanced Cognitive Function: Chair yoga involves mindfulness practices that can improve cognitive function and mental clarity in seniors. By focusing on the present moment and coordinating movement with breath, seniors can sharpen their attention and concentration.

14. Pain Management: For seniors dealing with chronic pain conditions like arthritis or fibromyalgia, chair yoga offers gentle movements and stretches that can help manage pain and improve overall comfort levels.

15. Increased Energy Levels: Chair yoga can boost seniors' energy levels by stimulating circulation, releasing tension, and promoting relaxation. Regular practice can lead to increased vitality and a greater sense of well-being throughout the day.

16. Supports Rehabilitation: Chair yoga can be an effective complement to traditional rehabilitation programs for seniors recovering from injuries, surgeries, or strokes. It provides a gentle yet effective way to regain strength, mobility, and confidence in movement.

17. Enhanced Digestion: Certain chair yoga poses and movements, particularly those that involve gentle twists and forward bends, can aid digestion and relieve symptoms of indigestion or constipation commonly experienced by seniors.

18. Emotional Well-being: Chair yoga promotes emotional well-being by reducing stress hormones like cortisol, increasing feel-good hormones like endorphins, and fostering a sense of relaxation and contentment among seniors.

19. Lifelong Learning: Chair yoga classes often incorporate elements of education and learning about the body, breath, and mindfulness practices. This lifelong learning aspect can stimulate seniors' curiosity, creativity, and cognitive engagement.

20. Adaptability and Empowerment: Chair yoga empowers seniors by providing them with tools and techniques they can use to manage their health and well-being independently. It promotes a sense of self-reliance and adaptability, empowering seniors to stay active and engaged in their daily lives.

21. Pain Prevention: In addition to managing existing pain, chair yoga can also help prevent future discomfort by improving posture, alignment, and muscle support, thus reducing the risk of developing musculoskeletal issues.

22. Joint Health: Chair yoga gently moves the joints through their full range of motion, promoting joint health and flexibility. This can be particularly beneficial for seniors with conditions like osteoarthritis or rheumatoid arthritis.

23. Heart Health: Some chair yoga sequences incorporate gentle cardiovascular exercises that can improve heart health, lower blood pressure, and reduce the risk of cardiovascular diseases in seniors.

24. Weight Management: Chair yoga, when combined with mindful eating habits and other lifestyle factors, can support weight management in seniors by increasing metabolism, promoting digestion, and burning calories.

25. Immune System Support: Regular practice of chair yoga can help support the immune system in seniors by reducing stress, promoting relaxation, and enhancing overall well-being, which are all factors known to contribute to a strong immune response.

26. Complementary Therapy: Chair yoga can be used as a complementary therapy alongside traditional medical treatments for various health conditions, providing seniors with a holistic approach to managing their health and well-being.

27. Improved Confidence: As seniors gain strength, flexibility, and balance through chair yoga practice, they often experience increased confidence in their physical abilities, leading to a greater sense of independence and self-assurance.

28. Creative Expression: Chair yoga classes sometimes incorporate creative elements such as visualization exercises, guided imagery, or expressive movements, providing seniors with opportunities for artistic expression and self-discovery.

29. Environmental Awareness: Chair yoga encourages seniors to develop a greater awareness of their physical environment, including the space around them and how their body interacts with it, fostering a deeper connection to their surroundings.

30. Spiritual Connection: For seniors who are interested in the spiritual aspects of yoga, chair yoga can provide opportunities for reflection, introspection, and inner exploration, leading to a greater sense of spiritual connection and fulfillment.

How to Use This Book

Title: Chair Yoga for Weight Loss for Seniors Over 60: A Comprehensive Guide to Wellness and Vitality

Welcome to "Chair Yoga for Weight Loss for Seniors Over 60"! This book is designed to be your comprehensive guide to achieving wellness and vitality through the practice of chair yoga. Whether you're a beginner or have some experience with yoga, this book will provide you with practical tips, step-by-step instructions, and motivating insights to help you on your journey towards weight loss and overall well-being.

Here's how to make the most of this book:

1. Get Started: Begin by familiarizing yourself with the introduction and overview of chair yoga. Learn about its benefits, principles, and how it can specifically support weight loss for seniors over 60.

2. Understand the Basics: Dive into the fundamentals of chair yoga, including proper posture, breathing techniques, and alignment principles. These basics are essential for a safe and effective practice.

3. Follow the Sequences: Explore a variety of chair yoga sequences specifically designed to promote weight loss and enhance overall fitness. Each sequence is accompanied by detailed instructions and illustrations to guide you through the poses and movements.

4. Embrace Mindful Eating: Discover how mindfulness can support your weight loss journey by promoting conscious eating habits and fostering a healthy relationship with food. Learn practical tips for incorporating mindful eating into your daily life.

5. Set Realistic Goals: Develop a personalized weight loss plan that aligns with your goals, preferences, and lifestyle. Use the goal-setting exercises provided in the book to define clear objectives and track your progress along the way.

6. Stay Motivated: Find inspiration and encouragement through motivational quotes, success stories, and tips for overcoming common challenges. Cultivate a positive mindset and stay committed to your journey towards better health and vitality.

7. Practice Self-Care: Remember to prioritize self-care as you embark on your weight loss journey. Explore relaxation techniques, stress management strategies, and tips for maintaining balance and well-being in all aspects of your life.

8. Create Your Routine: Develop a consistent chair yoga practice that fits seamlessly into your daily routine. Use the sample schedules and customizable workout plans provided in the book to create a routine that works for you.

9. Track Your Progress: Keep track of your achievements, milestones, and improvements along the way. Use the progress tracker and journaling prompts included in the book to reflect on your journey and celebrate your successes.

10. Seek Support: Connect with a community of like-minded individuals who share your goals and aspirations. Join online forums, attend local classes, or form a support group to stay motivated and accountable.

11. Nutritional Guidance: In addition to chair yoga sequences and mindfulness practices, this book provides valuable nutritional guidance tailored specifically for seniors over 60 who are looking to lose weight. Learn about healthy eating habits, portion control, and nutrient-rich foods that can support your weight loss goals.

12. Adaptability and Accessibility: One of the key features of this book is its focus on adaptability and accessibility. Chair yoga poses and sequences are carefully selected and modified to suit seniors of all fitness levels and physical abilities. Whether you're new to yoga or have limited mobility, you'll find options that work for you.

13. Progressive Approach: "Chair Yoga for Weight Loss for Seniors Over 60" takes a progressive approach to help readers gradually build strength, flexibility, and endurance over time. Each chapter builds upon the previous one, allowing you to advance at your own pace and steadily progress towards your weight loss goals.

14. Holistic Wellness: While weight loss is a central focus of this book, it also emphasizes holistic wellness and the importance of nurturing your mind, body, and spirit. Explore additional topics such as stress management, sleep hygiene, and self-care practices that contribute to overall well-being.

15. Personal Transformation: Beyond physical changes, "Chair Yoga for Weight Loss for Seniors Over 60" encourages readers to embrace a mindset of personal transformation. Discover how chair yoga can help you cultivate self-awareness, self-acceptance, and a positive body image as you embark on your weight loss journey.

16. Long-Term Success Strategies: This book doesn't just offer quick fixes or temporary solutions; it provides readers with long-term success strategies for sustainable weight loss and

lifestyle changes. Learn how to set realistic goals, overcome obstacles, and maintain your progress for the long haul.

17. Comprehensive Resource: Consider "Chair Yoga for Weight Loss for Seniors Over 60" as your go-to resource for all things related to chair yoga, weight loss, and senior fitness. Whether you're looking for specific poses, meal planning tips, or motivation to stay on track, you'll find it all within these pages.

18. Interactive Elements: Engage with the material in a meaningful way through interactive elements such as reflection questions, journaling prompts, and self-assessment tools. These interactive features encourage introspection, self-discovery, and personal growth throughout your weight loss journey.

19. Professional Guidance: Rest assured that the information and guidance provided in this book are backed by professional expertise and experience. The author, a certified yoga instructor specializing in senior fitness and weight loss, shares her knowledge and insights to help you achieve your goals safely and effectively.

20. Community Support: Finally, "Chair Yoga for Weight Loss for Seniors Over 60" fosters a sense of community and support among readers. Connect with others who are on similar journeys through online forums, social media groups, and virtual events organized by the author or other members of the chair yoga community.

With "Chair Yoga for Weight Loss for Seniors Over 60" as your guide, you'll have everything you need to embark on a transformative journey towards better health, vitality, and well-being. Let the journey begin!

Chapter 1: Getting Started with Chair Yoga

Understanding Chair Yoga:

Chair yoga is a gentle form of yoga that adapts traditional yoga poses and techniques to be performed while sitting on a chair or using a chair for support. It is designed to make yoga accessible to individuals who may have mobility issues, balance concerns, or difficulty getting up and down from the floor, such as seniors, people with disabilities, or those recovering from injuries.

Key Elements of Chair Yoga:

1. Seated Poses: Chair yoga focuses on a variety of seated poses that target different muscle groups and promote flexibility, strength, and balance. These poses can be modified to accommodate individual needs and abilities.

2. Breathing Exercises: Chair yoga incorporates breathing techniques (pranayama) to promote relaxation, reduce stress, and increase oxygen flow to the body. These exercises are particularly beneficial for seniors and individuals with respiratory conditions.

3. Mindfulness and Meditation: Chair yoga often includes elements of mindfulness and meditation to enhance mental clarity, focus, and emotional well-being. Participants are encouraged to cultivate awareness of their breath, body sensations, and thoughts.

4. Adaptability: One of the defining features of chair yoga is its adaptability. Practitioners can adjust the intensity of poses, use props for support, or choose alternative movements to accommodate physical limitations or health concerns.

5. Inclusivity: Chair yoga is inclusive and welcoming to people of all ages, fitness levels, and physical abilities. It provides a safe and supportive environment for individuals who may feel intimidated or excluded from traditional yoga classes.

<u>Benefits of Chair Yoga:</u>

1. Improved Flexibility and Range of Motion: Chair yoga helps improve flexibility by gently stretching muscles and joints, promoting mobility and range of motion.

2. Enhanced Strength: Through seated poses and resistance exercises, chair yoga helps build and maintain muscle strength, which is important for functional movements and balance.

3. Better Posture: Chair yoga emphasizes proper alignment and body awareness, helping improve posture and reduce strain on the spine and joints.

4. Stress Reduction: Breathing exercises and relaxation techniques in chair yoga promote stress reduction, leading to a greater sense of calm and well-being.

5. Pain Management: Chair yoga can help alleviate chronic pain conditions by gently stretching and strengthening muscles, promoting circulation, and reducing tension.

6. Improved Mental Health: Mindfulness practices in chair yoga can enhance mental clarity, focus, and emotional resilience, contributing to overall mental health and well-being.

7. Community and Social Connection: Chair yoga classes provide an opportunity for social interaction and connection, reducing feelings of isolation and fostering a sense of community among participants.

8. Accessibility: Chair yoga is highly accessible, making it suitable for individuals with a wide range of physical abilities and conditions. Whether someone is recovering from an injury, managing chronic pain, or dealing with mobility limitations, chair yoga can be adapted to meet their needs. This inclusivity allows more people to experience the benefits of yoga without feeling intimidated or discouraged by physical challenges.

9. Safety: Chair yoga prioritizes safety by providing support and stability throughout the practice. The chair serves as a prop for balance and assistance, reducing the risk of falls or injury, especially for seniors or those with balance issues. Additionally, the seated position minimizes strain on the joints and spine, making it a gentle and safe option for those with physical limitations or injuries.

10. Convenience: Chair yoga can be practiced virtually anywhere, making it convenient for individuals to incorporate into their daily lives. Whether at home, in the office, or during travel, all that's needed is a chair and some space. This accessibility eliminates barriers to consistent practice, allowing individuals to reap the benefits of yoga without the need for specialized equipment or dedicated studio space.

11. Relaxation and Stress Relief: Chair yoga offers relaxation techniques that can help reduce stress and promote a sense of calm and well-being. Breathing exercises, guided relaxation, and mindfulness practices incorporated into chair yoga sessions can help individuals unwind, release tension, and cultivate a greater sense of relaxation amidst the demands of daily life.

12. Improved Circulation and Digestion: The gentle movements and stretches of chair yoga can promote better circulation and digestion. By stimulating blood flow and encouraging movement in the muscles and joints, chair yoga can alleviate stiffness, improve digestion, and support overall cardiovascular health.

13. Enhanced Body Awareness: Chair yoga encourages participants to cultivate greater body awareness, mindfulness, and self-compassion. Through focused attention on breath and movement, individuals can deepen their connection to their bodies, become more attuned to physical sensations, and develop a greater sense of self-care and self-acceptance.

14. Adaptability for Chronic Conditions: Chair yoga can be adapted to accommodate various chronic conditions, such as arthritis, osteoporosis, or fibromyalgia. Modifications to poses and

movements can be made to address specific needs and limitations, allowing individuals to participate safely and comfortably while still experiencing the benefits of yoga.

15. Complementary Therapy: Chair yoga can complement other forms of therapy or treatment for various health conditions. Whether as a standalone practice or in conjunction with physical therapy, occupational therapy, or mental health counseling, chair yoga can support overall well-being and contribute to a holistic approach to health and healing.

Choosing the Right Equipment

When selecting equipment for chair yoga aimed at weight loss for seniors over 60, it's important to prioritize safety, comfort, and accessibility. Here are some considerations:

1. Sturdy Chairs: Choose chairs that are sturdy and stable to support the weight of the individuals. Armless chairs with a straight back and no wheels are ideal to ensure proper alignment during poses.

2. Comfortable Cushions: Provide cushions or pillows to support individuals with limited mobility or discomfort. These can be used to elevate the hips or support the lower back during seated poses.

3. Resistance Bands: Incorporate resistance bands to add strength training elements to the practice. These bands can be used for arm exercises, leg lifts, and stretching routines to enhance muscle tone and aid in weight loss.

4. Light Weights: Consider using light weights or resistance balls to add resistance and intensity to exercises without putting too much strain on joints. These can be incorporated into seated poses for added challenge.

5. Yoga Straps: Yoga straps can assist individuals with limited flexibility to achieve proper alignment in poses. They can also be used for gentle stretching exercises to improve flexibility and mobility.

6. Water Bottles: Encourage hydration during the practice by providing water bottles within reach. Staying hydrated is important for overall health and can support weight loss efforts.

7. Non-Slip Mats: If practicing standing poses or balance exercises, use non-slip mats to prevent slips and falls. Safety should always be a priority, especially for seniors.

8. Instructional Materials: Provide instructional materials such as posters or handouts demonstrating poses and modifications tailored for seniors. Clear instructions and visual aids can help participants understand and execute poses correctly.

9. Adjustable Height Blocks: Use adjustable height blocks to accommodate individuals with varying levels of flexibility. These blocks can provide support during seated poses or serve as props for modifications.

10. Music and Relaxation Tools: Consider incorporating soothing music or relaxation tools such as meditation apps or guided imagery to enhance the overall experience and promote relaxation, which can support weight loss goals by reducing stress levels.

11. Chair Modifications: Ensure that the chairs used for chair yoga are adjustable to accommodate different body sizes and mobility levels. Consider using chairs with removable armrests or seats that can be raised or lowered to provide optimal support and comfort for participants.

12. Ankle Weights: Integrate ankle weights into the practice to add resistance to lower body exercises such as leg lifts and ankle circles. Ankle weights can help increase muscle engagement and calorie burn during seated or standing poses, contributing to weight loss goals.

13. Therapeutic Balls: Incorporate small therapeutic balls or massage balls into the practice to release tension and improve circulation. Participants can use these balls to perform self-massage techniques on areas of tightness or discomfort, promoting relaxation and aiding in weight loss through stress reduction.

14. Visual Props: Utilize visual props such as mirrors or demonstration videos to assist participants in understanding and executing poses correctly. Visual aids can help seniors over 60 maintain proper alignment and form, maximizing the effectiveness of their chair yoga practice for weight loss.

15. Temperature Control: Ensure that the practice space is adequately ventilated and maintained at a comfortable temperature for participants. Consider using fans or air conditioning to prevent overheating during physical activity, especially for seniors who may be more sensitive to temperature changes.

16. Accessibility Aids: Provide accessibility aids such as handrails or support bars near chairs to assist participants with balance or mobility challenges. These aids can enhance safety and confidence during chair yoga practice, enabling seniors over 60 to engage more fully in their weight loss journey.

17. Educational Resources: Offer educational resources such as books, articles, or workshops on nutrition and healthy eating habits to complement the physical practice of chair yoga. Encouraging participants to make dietary changes alongside their yoga practice can support their weight loss goals and overall well-being.

18. Community Support: Foster a sense of community and support among participants by organizing group activities or social events related to chair yoga and weight loss. Providing opportunities for seniors over 60 to connect with peers who share similar goals can enhance motivation and accountability on their wellness journey.

<u>Safety Precautions and Modifications</u>

When practicing chair yoga for weight loss as a senior, safety precautions and modifications are crucial. Here are some key points to consider:

1. Consult with a healthcare professional: Before starting any exercise program, especially if you have existing health conditions or concerns, it's essential to consult with your healthcare provider to ensure chair yoga is safe for you.

2. Use a sturdy chair: Choose a stable chair without wheels, preferably with a straight back and no arms. This provides better support and stability during poses.

3. Warm-up: Begin each session with a gentle warm-up to prepare your body for movement. This can include simple neck, shoulder, and wrist rotations, as well as deep breathing exercises.

4. Listen to your body: Pay attention to how your body feels during each pose. If you experience pain or discomfort, ease out of the pose immediately and modify as needed.

5. Modify poses: Many traditional yoga poses can be adapted for chair yoga. For example, instead of standing forward fold, you can do a seated forward fold by gently bending forward from the hips while seated on the chair.

6. Focus on alignment: Proper alignment is crucial to prevent injury and maximize the benefits of each pose. Engage your core muscles, maintain a straight spine, and avoid overextending or straining.

7. Breath awareness: Coordinate your breath with movement to enhance relaxation and mindfulness. Practice deep, controlled breathing throughout the session.

8. Stay hydrated: Drink water before, during, and after your practice to stay hydrated, especially if you're sweating.

9.*Gradually increase intensity: Start with gentle poses and gradually increase the intensity and duration of your practice as your strength and flexibility improve.

10. Cool down: End each session with a few minutes of relaxation and deep breathing to allow your body to rest and recover.

Importance of Breathing in Yoga

The importance of breathing in yoga cannot be overstated, as it serves as the cornerstone of the practice, linking the physical, mental, and spiritual aspects of our being. In yoga philosophy, the breath is referred to as "prana," or life force energy, and is considered the bridge between the body and the mind. By cultivating awareness of the breath during yoga practice, practitioners tap into this vital energy, allowing it to flow freely throughout the body, revitalizing cells, and nourishing tissues. Conscious breathing techniques, known as "pranayama," are integral to yoga practice, offering a myriad of benefits for physical, mental, and emotional well-being. Deep, diaphragmatic breathing improves lung capacity, enhances respiratory function, and oxygenates the blood, promoting overall vitality and health. Moreover, breath-focused practices regulate the autonomic nervous system, balancing the body's stress response and inducing a state of relaxation and calmness. This, in turn, reduces stress levels, lowers blood pressure, and boosts the immune system. Beyond the physical realm, mindful breathing cultivates mental clarity, concentration, and presence, anchoring the mind in the present moment and quieting mental chatter. It also serves as a tool for emotional regulation, allowing practitioners to navigate challenges with resilience and equanimity. Ultimately, the importance of breathing in yoga extends beyond the mat, permeating every aspect of our lives, fostering a deeper connection with ourselves and the world around us. Through conscious breath awareness, we tap into the essence of our being, awakening to the boundless potential within and embracing the journey of self-discovery and transformation.

The importance of breathing in yoga cannot be overstated, as it is considered the foundation of the practice. Here's why:

1. Mind-body connection: Breath is the bridge between the mind and body in yoga. Focusing on the breath allows practitioners to cultivate mindfulness and awareness of their physical sensations, thoughts, and emotions during practice.

2. Stress reduction: Conscious breathing techniques, such as deep breathing or diaphragmatic breathing, activate the parasympathetic nervous system, which promotes relaxation and reduces stress levels. This is particularly beneficial in today's fast-paced world, where stress is prevalent.

3. Energy regulation: Pranayama, or breath control techniques, are an integral part of yoga practice. Different pranayama techniques can either energize the body or induce relaxation, helping to balance and regulate the body's energy levels.

4. Improves focus and concentration: Deep, mindful breathing anchors the mind in the present moment, enhancing focus and concentration during yoga practice. This heightened awareness can lead to a deeper connection with the body and a more profound experience on the mat.

5. Enhances physical performance: Coordinating movement with breath in yoga sequences improves coordination, balance, and proprioception. The breath provides a rhythm and pace to the practice, allowing practitioners to move more gracefully and efficiently through poses.

6. Supports detoxification: Deep breathing aids in the removal of toxins from the body by increasing oxygenation and circulation. This supports the body's natural detoxification processes and promotes overall health and well-being.

7. Stimulates relaxation response: Controlled breathing activates the body's relaxation response, which can help alleviate symptoms of anxiety, depression, and insomnia. Regular practice of breath-focused yoga techniques can improve sleep quality and promote emotional balance.

8. Cultivates mindfulness: Breath awareness is a fundamental aspect of mindfulness practice. By tuning into the breath during yoga, practitioners learn to observe their thoughts and physical sensations without judgment, fostering a sense of inner peace and acceptance.

9. Improves respiratory function: Yoga breathing techniques, or pranayama, focus on deepening and expanding the breath. Regular practice can improve lung capacity, strengthen respiratory muscles, and enhance overall respiratory function. This is particularly beneficial for individuals with respiratory conditions such as asthma or chronic obstructive pulmonary disease (COPD).

10. Promotes emotional balance: The breath is intimately connected to our emotions. Shallow, rapid breathing is often associated with stress, anxiety, or fear, while slow, deep breathing induces feelings of calmness and relaxation. By consciously regulating the breath through yoga, practitioners can cultivate emotional balance and resilience, reducing the impact of negative emotions on their well-being.

11. Increases body awareness: Paying attention to the breath during yoga practice enhances body awareness and proprioception, which is the sense of the body's position in space. This heightened

awareness allows practitioners to move more mindfully, aligning their movements with their breath and minimizing the risk of injury.

12. Balances the autonomic nervous system: The autonomic nervous system regulates involuntary bodily functions such as heart rate, digestion, and respiratory rate. Through breath-focused yoga practices, practitioners can influence the balance between the sympathetic nervous system (responsible for the "fight or flight" response) and the parasympathetic nervous system (responsible for rest and relaxation), promoting overall well-being and stress resilience.

13. Facilitates meditation: Breath awareness serves as a gateway to meditation in yoga practice. By anchoring the mind to the rhythmic flow of the breath, practitioners can enter a state of deep concentration and inner stillness, facilitating meditation and introspection. This meditative aspect of yoga fosters self-awareness, insight, and spiritual growth.

14. Enhances athletic performance: The breath plays a crucial role in athletic performance, including in activities beyond yoga. Controlled breathing techniques can help athletes optimize their performance by managing energy levels, reducing fatigue, and improving focus and concentration during physical exertion.

15. Supports overall well-being: Ultimately, the importance of breathing in yoga extends to promoting holistic well-being – encompassing physical, mental, emotional, and spiritual aspects of health. By cultivating a deeper relationship with the breath through yoga practice, practitioners can experience greater vitality, resilience, and harmony in their lives.

16. Regulates the mind: Breath control in yoga, known as pranayama, directly influences the mind's fluctuations. Through specific breathing techniques, practitioners can calm an agitated mind, sharpen focus, and cultivate mental clarity. This regulation of the mind is integral to achieving deeper states of meditation and self-awareness.

17. Supports emotional release: The breath serves as a bridge between the conscious and subconscious mind. During yoga practice, conscious breathing can bring awareness to suppressed emotions and tensions stored in the body. Through mindful breathing, practitioners can gently release emotional blockages, leading to a sense of emotional liberation and inner peace.

18. Promotes mindfulness off the mat: The mindfulness cultivated through breath-centered yoga practice extends beyond the mat into daily life. By learning to anchor attention to the breath during challenging situations, practitioners can respond to stressors with greater resilience, equanimity, and presence, fostering a more mindful and balanced lifestyle.

19. Enhances circulation and oxygenation: Deep, diaphragmatic breathing improves circulation and oxygenation throughout the body. Oxygen-rich blood nourishes cells, supports tissue repair, and enhances overall vitality. By consciously deepening the breath during yoga practice, practitioners optimize the body's physiological functions, promoting health and vitality.

20. Facilitates energetic balance: According to yoga philosophy, prana, or life force energy, flows through the breath. Through pranayama practices, practitioners can regulate and balance the flow of prana within the subtle energy channels (nadis) and energy centers (chakras) of the body. This energetic balance promotes physical, mental, and emotional well-being.

21. Deepens self-awareness: The breath serves as a mirror reflecting our inner state. By observing the quality and pattern of the breath during yoga practice, practitioners gain insight into their physical, mental, and emotional states. This heightened self-awareness allows for greater self-understanding and facilitates personal growth and transformation.

22. Connects to the present moment: The breath is inherently linked to the present moment, as it can only be experienced in the here and now. By anchoring attention to the breath during yoga practice, practitioners cultivate mindfulness and presence, letting go of regrets about the past and worries about the future. This present-moment awareness fosters a deep sense of peace and contentment.

23. Promotes longevity: Deep, conscious breathing has been associated with longevity and vitality in various spiritual and cultural traditions. By incorporating breath-centered yoga practices into daily life, practitioners not only enhance their physical and mental well-being but also cultivate a profound sense of vitality and longevity.

In summary, the importance of breathing in yoga extends far beyond the physical act of inhaling and exhaling. It influences every aspect of our being – from physical health and emotional well-being to mental clarity and spiritual growth.

Chair Yoga Breathing Exercises

Chair yoga breathing exercises are accessible and beneficial for individuals of all ages and abilities. Here are some chair yoga breathing exercises you can incorporate into your practice:

1. Seated Deep Breathing: Sit comfortably in a chair with your feet flat on the ground and your hands resting on your thighs. Close your eyes or soften your gaze. Inhale deeply through your nose, expanding your belly as you fill your lungs with air. Exhale slowly and completely through your nose or mouth, emptying your lungs and drawing your belly button towards your spine. Repeat for several breaths, focusing on the sensation of the breath moving in and out of your body.

2. Three-Part Breath: Sit tall in your chair with your feet flat on the ground and your hands resting on your abdomen. Inhale deeply through your nose, first filling your lower belly, then your ribcage, and finally your chest. Exhale slowly and completely, releasing the breath from your chest, then your ribcage, and finally your lower belly. Repeat this three-part breath for several cycles, maintaining a smooth and continuous flow.

3. Counted Breathing: Sit comfortably in your chair and close your eyes or soften your gaze. Inhale deeply through your nose to a count of four, then hold your breath for a count of four.

Exhale slowly and completely through your nose or mouth to a count of four, and then hold your breath for a count of four before beginning the next cycle. Repeat for several rounds, gradually increasing the count if comfortable.

4. Alternate Nostril Breathing: Sit comfortably with your spine tall and your feet flat on the ground. Rest your left hand on your left knee or thigh. With your right hand, bring your index and middle fingers to your forehead, resting lightly on the space between your eyebrows. Use your thumb to close your right nostril and your ring finger or pinky to close your left nostril. Begin by closing your right nostril and inhaling deeply through your left nostril. Close your left nostril with your ring finger or pinky and exhale through your right nostril. Inhale deeply through your right nostril, then close it with your thumb and exhale through your left nostril. Continue this alternate nostril breathing for several rounds, maintaining a slow and steady breath.

5. Bee's Breath (Bhramari Pranayama): Sit comfortably in your chair with your spine tall and your hands resting on your thighs. Close your eyes or soften your gaze. Inhale deeply through your nose, and as you exhale, make a gentle humming sound like a bee, keeping your lips lightly closed and the back of your throat slightly constricted. Allow the sound to be smooth, steady, and soothing. Repeat for several rounds, focusing on the vibrations and calming effect of the sound.

6. Abdominal Breathing with Visualization: Sit comfortably in your chair with your feet flat on the ground and your hands resting on your abdomen. Close your eyes or soften your gaze. Inhale deeply through your nose, allowing your abdomen to expand like a balloon. As you exhale, visualize releasing any tension or stress from your body, allowing it to dissolve with each breath

out. Continue this abdominal breathing with visualization for several cycles, focusing on the soothing rhythm of your breath and the calming imagery.

7. Box Breathing: Sit tall in your chair with your feet flat on the ground and your hands resting on your thighs. Close your eyes or soften your gaze. Inhale deeply through your nose to a count of four, feeling the breath fill your lungs completely. Hold your breath for a count of four, maintaining a sense of stillness and presence. Exhale slowly and completely through your nose or mouth to a count of four, releasing any tension or tightness from your body. Hold your breath out for a count of four before beginning the next cycle. Repeat this box breathing pattern for several rounds, focusing on the equal length of each breath phase and the sense of balance it brings.

8. Extended Exhalation: Sit comfortably in your chair with your feet flat on the ground and your hands resting on your thighs. Close your eyes or soften your gaze. Inhale deeply through your nose to a count of three or four, filling your lungs with air. Exhale slowly and completely through your nose or mouth to a count of six or eight, allowing your breath to extend longer than the inhale. Repeat this extended exhalation for several cycles, focusing on the calming and grounding effect it has on your body and mind.

9. Cleansing Breath (Kapalabhati Pranayama): Sit tall in your chair with your feet flat on the ground and your hands resting on your thighs. Close your eyes or soften your gaze. Take a deep inhalation through your nose, filling your lungs with air. Exhale forcefully and rapidly through your nose, engaging your abdominal muscles to push the breath out in short bursts. Allow the

inhalation to happen passively as your abdomen naturally expands. Repeat this rapid exhalation for several rounds, followed by a few deep, calming breaths to return to a state of relaxation.

10. Gratitude Breath: Sit comfortably in your chair with your feet flat on the ground and your hands resting on your thighs. Close your eyes or soften your gaze. Take a moment to reflect on something you're grateful for in your life. As you inhale deeply through your nose, silently repeat the word "gratitude" or a related affirmation to yourself. As you exhale slowly and completely through your nose or mouth, visualize sending feelings of gratitude and appreciation out into the world. Repeat this gratitude breath for several cycles, allowing each inhale to fill you with a sense of thankfulness and each exhale to share that gratitude with others.

11. Sama Vritti (Equal Breathing): Sit comfortably in your chair with your feet flat on the ground and your hands resting on your thighs. Close your eyes or soften your gaze. Inhale deeply through your nose to a count of four, and then exhale through your nose to the same count of four. Keep the inhale and exhale equal in length, maintaining a smooth and steady rhythm. Continue this equal breathing pattern for several rounds, focusing on the sensation of balance and harmony with each breath cycle.

12. Progressive Relaxation Breathing: Sit comfortably in your chair with your feet flat on the ground and your hands resting on your thighs. Close your eyes or soften your gaze. Begin by tensing the muscles in your feet and toes as you inhale deeply through your nose. Hold the tension for a few seconds, and then exhale slowly as you release the tension from your feet and toes. Move sequentially through each muscle group in your body, tensing and releasing as you

breathe deeply. Continue this progressive relaxation breathing, moving from your feet all the way up to your head and neck, allowing your body to soften and relax with each exhalation.

13. Visualization Breath: Sit comfortably in your chair with your feet flat on the ground and your hands resting on your thighs. Close your eyes or soften your gaze. As you inhale deeply through your nose, visualize drawing in positive energy, light, or a sense of peace and calmness. As you exhale slowly and completely through your nose or mouth, visualize releasing any tension, stress, or negative thoughts from your body and mind. Repeat this visualization breath for several cycles, focusing on the imagery and sensations you cultivate with each breath.

14. Ujjayi Breathing (Ocean Breath): Sit comfortably in your chair with your feet flat on the ground and your hands resting on your thighs. Close your eyes or soften your gaze. Inhale deeply through your nose, and then exhale slowly and completely through your nose, slightly constricting the back of your throat to create a soft, audible sound like the ocean waves. Allow the sound of your breath to be smooth and steady, like the rhythmic ebb and flow of the tide. Continue this ujjayi breathing for several rounds, allowing it to soothe your nervous system and bring a sense of calmness and tranquility.

15. Pursed Lip Breathing: Sit comfortably in your chair with your feet flat on the ground and your hands resting on your thighs. Close your eyes or soften your gaze. Inhale deeply through your nose, and then exhale slowly and gently through pursed lips, as if you are blowing out a candle. Allow the exhale to be smooth and controlled, focusing on releasing tension from your

body and mind with each breath out. Repeat this pursed lip breathing for several cycles, noticing how it calms your nervous system and promotes relaxation.

16. Sitali Pranayama (Cooling Breath): Sit comfortably in your chair with your feet flat on the ground and your hands resting on your thighs. Close your eyes or soften your gaze. Curl your tongue into a "U" shape or purse your lips if you cannot curl your tongue. Inhale deeply through your curled tongue or pursed lips, allowing the breath to feel cool as it enters your mouth. Exhale slowly and completely through your nose. Repeat this cooling breath for several rounds, focusing on the sensation of coolness as you inhale and the warmth as you exhale.

17. Belly Breathing: Sit comfortably in your chair with your feet flat on the ground and your hands resting on your abdomen. Close your eyes or soften your gaze. Place one hand on your chest and the other on your abdomen. Inhale deeply through your nose, allowing your abdomen to rise as you fill your lungs with air. Feel your chest expand slightly. Exhale slowly and completely through your nose, feeling your abdomen gently fall as you empty your lungs. Focus on breathing deeply into your belly, allowing it to rise and fall with each breath cycle.

18. 4-7-8 Breathing: Sit comfortably in your chair with your feet flat on the ground and your hands resting on your thighs. Close your eyes or soften your gaze. Inhale deeply through your nose to a count of four. Hold your breath for a count of seven. Exhale slowly and completely through your mouth to a count of eight, making a whooshing sound as you release the breath. Repeat this 4-7-8 breathing pattern for several rounds, focusing on the elongated exhale and the calming effect it has on your nervous system.

19. Counted Breath Retention: Sit comfortably in your chair with your feet flat on the ground and your hands resting on your thighs. Close your eyes or soften your gaze. Inhale deeply through your nose to a count of four. Hold your breath for a count of four. Exhale slowly and completely through your nose or mouth to a count of four. Hold your breath out for a count of four. Repeat this counted breath retention for several rounds, focusing on the equal length of each phase of the breath and the sense of balance it brings.

Seated Forward Bend

The Seated Forward Bend, also known as Paschimottanasana in Sanskrit, is a popular chair yoga pose that offers numerous benefits, including aiding in weight loss. To perform this pose, sit comfortably on a chair with your feet flat on the ground and your spine tall. Inhale deeply to lengthen your spine, then exhale as you hinge forward from your hips, keeping your back straight. Lower your chest towards your thighs and reach your hands towards your feet or ankles, resting them wherever is comfortable for you. Keep your neck relaxed and avoid rounding your back. Hold this position for several breaths, feeling a gentle stretch along the back of your legs and spine. The Seated Forward Bend helps to stimulate digestion, improve metabolism, and activate the abdominal muscles, making it an effective pose for supporting weight loss efforts. Additionally, it promotes relaxation and relieves tension in the back and neck, enhancing overall well-being. Practice this pose regularly as part of your chair yoga routine to experience its weight loss benefits and improve flexibility in your spine and hamstrings.

The Seated Forward Bend (Paschimottanasana) is a foundational yoga pose that offers a multitude of benefits beyond weight loss. Here's a deeper exploration of its effects:

1. Stretches the spine and hamstrings: As you fold forward in the Seated Forward Bend, you lengthen and stretch the entire length of your spine, from the base of your spine (sacrum) to the crown of your head. This helps to alleviate tension and stiffness in the back, improve spinal flexibility, and promote better posture. Additionally, the pose stretches the hamstrings (the muscles at the back of your thighs), which can become tight from prolonged sitting or lack of movement.

2. Stimulates the digestive organs: The forward folding action of the Seated Forward Bend compresses the abdomen, stimulating the digestive organs, including the stomach, liver, pancreas, and intestines. This gentle compression can help improve digestion, relieve constipation, and alleviate bloating. By promoting healthy digestion, the pose supports overall digestive health, which is important for maintaining a healthy weight.

3. Calms the mind and relieves stress: The gentle, forward folding nature of the pose encourages relaxation and helps to calm the mind. As you focus on the breath and release tension in the body, the Seated Forward Bend can promote a sense of tranquility and mental clarity. This relaxation response can be beneficial for managing stress, anxiety, and emotional eating, which are often associated with weight management challenges.

4. Stimulates the urinary system: The compression of the abdomen in the Seated Forward Bend also stimulates the urinary system, including the kidneys and bladder. This can help improve urinary function and promote detoxification by encouraging the elimination of waste products and toxins from the body.

5. Improves circulation: The forward folding action in the Seated Forward Bend promotes blood flow to the brain, which can help improve concentration and mental alertness. Additionally, the pose can help alleviate symptoms of fatigue and sluggishness by increasing circulation throughout the body, leading to a feeling of rejuvenation and vitality.

6. Modifications for accessibility: The Seated Forward Bend can be easily modified to accommodate different levels of flexibility and mobility. For example, if you have tight hamstrings or limited flexibility in the spine, you can use props such as a yoga strap or belt to loop around your feet and provide support as you fold forward. Additionally, you can perform a seated version of the pose by sitting on the edge of a chair and folding forward with your hands resting on your thighs.

Spinal Twist

The Spinal Twist is a popular chair yoga pose that offers numerous benefits, including promoting flexibility, improving digestion, and supporting weight loss goals. To perform the Spinal Twist while seated in a chair, begin by sitting tall with your feet flat on the ground and your hands resting on your thighs. Take a deep breath in to lengthen your spine, and as you exhale, twist your torso to the right, placing your left hand on the outside of your right thigh and your right hand on the back of the chair. Use your hands to gently deepen the twist, taking care not to strain. Hold the twist for several breaths, feeling the stretch along the spine and through the waist. On an inhale, return to center, and then exhale as you twist to the left, placing your right hand on the outside of your left thigh and your left hand on the back of the chair. Again, use your hands to deepen the twist, breathing deeply and holding the pose for several breaths. The Spinal Twist helps to stimulate digestion, release tension in the back and shoulders, and improve spinal mobility, all of which can support weight loss efforts. Incorporate this gentle twist into your chair yoga practice to experience its rejuvenating benefits for body and mind.

The Spinal Twist is a versatile chair yoga pose that offers a wide range of benefits beyond weight loss. Here are some additional details about this pose:

1. Improved Digestion: The twisting motion of the Spinal Twist stimulates the abdominal organs, including the digestive organs. This can help improve digestion and alleviate digestive discomfort such as bloating and gas, which are common obstacles to weight loss.

2. Detoxification: Twisting poses like the Spinal Twist can aid in detoxification by wringing out toxins from the organs and tissues. As you twist, you create space in the abdomen, allowing for better circulation and lymphatic drainage, which supports the body's natural detoxification processes.

3. Enhanced Spinal Mobility: The Spinal Twist stretches and strengthens the muscles along the spine, promoting spinal mobility and flexibility. This can help alleviate stiffness and discomfort in the back, neck, and shoulders, which may result from sedentary lifestyles or poor posture, ultimately supporting better overall movement and posture.

4. Stress Reduction: Twisting poses in yoga are known for their calming and grounding effects on the nervous system. The gentle compression of the abdomen in the Spinal Twist can help activate the parasympathetic nervous system, promoting relaxation and reducing stress levels. Lowering stress levels can be beneficial for weight loss by reducing the production of stress hormones like cortisol, which can contribute to weight gain.

5. Improved Circulation: Twisting poses like the Spinal Twist can also help improve circulation throughout the body. As you twist, you create a compression and release effect on the muscles

and tissues, which can help enhance blood flow and oxygenation to the organs and extremities. Improved circulation supports overall health and vitality, which can aid in weight loss efforts.

6. Mind-Body Connection: The Spinal Twist encourages practitioners to focus on their breath and body awareness, fostering a deeper connection between the mind and body. This mindfulness practice can help cultivate a sense of presence and awareness during the pose, which can translate into mindful eating habits and greater self-awareness, supporting overall well-being and weight management.

Cat-Cow Stretch

The Cat-Cow Stretch is a gentle and effective chair yoga pose that can aid in weight loss by promoting flexibility, mobility, and circulation throughout the spine and torso. To perform the Cat-Cow Stretch in a chair, begin by sitting comfortably with your feet flat on the ground and your hands resting on your thighs. Inhale deeply as you arch your back, lifting your chest and gaze towards the ceiling while gently pulling your shoulders back. This is the "Cow" phase of the stretch, which stretches the front of the torso and opens the chest, promoting better posture and lung capacity. Exhale slowly as you round your spine, tucking your chin towards your chest and drawing your navel towards your spine. This is the "Cat" phase of the stretch, which engages the abdominal muscles and stretches the back of the torso, promoting spinal flexibility and core strength. Flow smoothly between the Cat and Cow phases, synchronizing your breath with movement for several rounds. This gentle dynamic movement helps to increase circulation, massage the internal organs, and release tension in the spine, which can aid in digestion and metabolism. Practicing the Cat-Cow Stretch regularly as part of a chair yoga routine can contribute to overall weight loss goals by promoting better posture, spinal health, and mindful movement throughout the body.

Here's some additional information on the Cat-Cow Stretch in chair yoga for weight loss:

1. Spinal Mobility: The Cat-Cow Stretch is particularly beneficial for improving spinal mobility, which is essential for overall movement and function. As you flow between the arching and rounding of the spine, you gently stretch and mobilize the vertebrae, helping to maintain flexibility and prevent stiffness in the spine. This increased mobility can enhance your ability to perform other physical activities, leading to greater calorie expenditure and weight loss over time.

2. Core Activation: While performing the Cat-Cow Stretch, you engage the muscles of the core, including the abdominals and obliques. This engagement helps to stabilize the spine and pelvis, improving posture and providing a foundation for other movements. Strengthening the core muscles through regular practice of the Cat-Cow Stretch can contribute to a stronger and more toned midsection, which can support weight loss efforts by increasing overall muscle mass and metabolism.

3. Breath Awareness: The Cat-Cow Stretch emphasizes coordinating movement with breath, which enhances breath awareness and mindfulness during the practice. Focusing on the breath helps to deepen the stretch, promote relaxation, and center the mind. This mindful breathing technique can reduce stress levels, improve mood, and support healthy eating habits, all of which are important factors in weight management and overall well-being.

4. Digestive Health: The gentle compression and release of the abdomen in the Cat-Cow Stretch can stimulate the digestive organs, promoting better digestion and nutrient absorption. A healthy digestive system is crucial for optimal metabolism and energy production, which are key components of successful weight loss. By incorporating the Cat-Cow Stretch into your chair yoga routine, you can support digestive health and improve overall nutrient utilization, contributing to your weight loss goals.

5. Mind-Body Connection: As with all yoga poses, the Cat-Cow Stretch encourages a deeper connection between the mind and body. By tuning into the sensations of the stretch and the rhythm of the breath, you cultivate greater body awareness and self-awareness. This heightened awareness can lead to more mindful eating habits, increased physical activity, and a greater sense of empowerment in your weight loss journey.

Warrior I and II in a Chair

Warrior I and II are dynamic yoga poses known for their ability to build strength, stability, and flexibility in the legs, hips, and core. While traditionally practiced standing, they can also be modified for chair yoga, making them accessible to individuals with limited mobility or those seeking a gentle yet effective workout for weight loss. Here's how to perform Warrior I and II in a chair:

1. Warrior I in a Chair: Begin by sitting tall in a sturdy chair with your feet hip-width apart and firmly planted on the ground. Extend your right leg straight back, keeping the toes pointing

forward and the heel lifted off the ground. Bend your left knee, ensuring it stays aligned with your ankle, and engage your core for stability. Inhale as you raise your arms overhead, reaching towards the ceiling with your fingertips. Square your hips towards the front of the chair and lift your chest, lengthening through the spine. Hold this pose for several breaths, focusing on grounding through the feet and lengthening through the torso. To release, exhale as you lower your arms and return your right foot to the ground. Repeat on the other side.

2. Warrior II in a Chair: From the seated position, extend your right leg straight out to the side, keeping the foot flat on the ground and the toes pointing forward. Bend your left knee, ensuring it stays aligned with your ankle, and open your hips towards the side of the chair. Inhale as you extend your arms out to the sides at shoulder height, parallel to the ground, with your palms facing down. Gaze over your left fingertips, keeping your shoulders relaxed and your chest lifted. Hold this pose for several breaths, focusing on grounding through the feet and maintaining stability in the lower body. To release, exhale as you lower your arms and return your right foot to the ground. Repeat on the other side.

Warrior I and II in a chair are powerful modifications of traditional yoga poses that offer numerous benefits for weight loss and overall fitness. Here are some additional details about these chair yoga poses:

1. Engagement of Core Muscles: Both Warrior I and II in a chair require engagement of the core muscles to maintain stability and balance. By activating the abdominal muscles, obliques, and lower back, these poses help strengthen the core, which is crucial for supporting the spine and improving posture. A strong core also aids in weight loss by promoting better alignment and efficiency in movement.

2. Strengthening of Lower Body: Warrior I and II in a chair target the muscles of the lower body, including the quadriceps, hamstrings, glutes, and calves. These poses help build strength and endurance in these muscle groups, which not only contributes to weight loss but also enhances overall physical performance and mobility. Stronger leg muscles can support activities of daily living and make other forms of exercise more accessible and effective.

3. Improvement of Flexibility: Practicing Warrior I and II in a chair can help improve flexibility in the hips, groin, and thighs. These poses require a deep stretch in the hip flexors, which can become tight and shortened due to prolonged periods of sitting. By regularly performing these chair yoga poses, individuals can increase their range of motion in the lower body, leading to greater ease of movement and reduced risk of injury.

4. Enhancement of Mental Focus: Like their standing counterparts, Warrior I and II in a chair require concentration and focus to maintain proper alignment and form. By directing attention to the breath and the sensations in the body during these poses, practitioners can cultivate mindfulness and present-moment awareness. This mental focus not only deepens the yoga practice but also promotes stress reduction and emotional well-being, which are essential components of successful weight loss journeys.

5. Adaptability for All Fitness Levels: One of the significant advantages of practicing Warrior I and II in a chair is their adaptability for individuals of all fitness levels and abilities. These poses can be modified to accommodate varying degrees of mobility, making them accessible to seniors,

individuals with mobility limitations, or those recovering from injuries. By providing a safe and supportive environment, chair yoga allows everyone to experience the benefits of these empowering poses.

Chair Pigeon Pose

Chair Pigeon Pose is a modified version of the traditional Pigeon Pose, adapted for chair yoga practice. It targets the hips, glutes, and lower back, making it an effective pose for stretching and strengthening these areas, which can contribute to weight loss by improving overall flexibility and mobility. To practice Chair Pigeon Pose, start by sitting comfortably in a chair with your feet flat on the ground and your spine tall. Cross your right ankle over your left knee, flexing your right foot to protect your knee joint. Keep your right knee in line with your right ankle to maintain proper alignment. You may feel a stretch in your right hip and glute. If you'd like to deepen the stretch, gently hinge forward from your hips while keeping your spine long, being mindful not to round your back. Hold the pose for several breaths, feeling the stretch deepen with each exhale. Then, switch sides by crossing your left ankle over your right knee and repeating the pose on the opposite side. Chair Pigeon Pose can be practiced regularly to improve hip flexibility, alleviate tension in the lower back, and promote overall relaxation, all of which support weight loss efforts by enhancing physical well-being and reducing stress levels.

Chair Pigeon Pose, also known as Seated Pigeon Pose or Chair Eka Pada Rajakapotasana in Sanskrit, is a beneficial chair yoga pose for weight loss that targets the hips, glutes, and lower back while providing a gentle stretch to the muscles and connective tissues. This pose is particularly beneficial for individuals with limited mobility or those who find traditional floor-based Pigeon Pose challenging.

To practice Chair Pigeon Pose, begin by sitting comfortably in a chair with your feet flat on the ground and your spine tall. Place your hands on your thighs for support. Then, cross your right ankle over your left knee, ensuring that your right knee is in line with your right ankle to protect the knee joint. Flex your right foot to engage the muscles of the leg and provide stability.

As you settle into the pose, you may feel a gentle stretch in your right hip and glute. If you'd like to deepen the stretch, you can gently hinge forward from your hips while maintaining a long spine. Be mindful not to round your back or strain your neck. Only go as far forward as feels comfortable for you, and remember to breathe deeply and evenly throughout the pose.

Hold Chair Pigeon Pose for several breaths, allowing the stretch to deepen with each exhale. Focus on relaxing any tension in the muscles and releasing any stress or tightness in the hips and lower back. After holding the pose for an appropriate amount of time, gently release and switch sides, crossing your left ankle over your right knee and repeating the pose on the opposite side.

Practicing Chair Pigeon Pose regularly can help improve hip flexibility, alleviate tension in the hips and lower back, and promote relaxation and stress relief. These benefits contribute to overall well-being and can support weight loss efforts by improving mobility, reducing discomfort, and enhancing the mind-body connection.

Morning Energizing Routine

A "Morning Energizing Routine" in chair yoga can be a fantastic way to start the day with vitality and positivity while also supporting weight loss goals. Here's a sample chair yoga routine designed to energize the body and mind:

1. Seated Cat-Cow Stretch: Begin by sitting comfortably in a chair with your feet flat on the ground and your hands resting on your thighs. Inhale as you arch your spine, lifting your chest and drawing your shoulder blades together (Cow Pose). Exhale as you round your spine, tucking your chin to your chest and drawing your navel towards your spine (Cat Pose). Flow smoothly between these two poses, coordinating your movements with your breath. Repeat for several rounds to warm up the spine and awaken the body.

2. Seated Side Stretch: Sit tall in your chair with your feet flat on the ground and your hands resting on your thighs. Inhale as you reach your right arm up towards the ceiling, lengthening through the right side of your body. Exhale as you gently lean to the left, feeling a stretch along the right side of your torso. Hold the stretch for a few breaths, then inhale to return to center. Repeat on the other side, reaching the left arm up and leaning to the right. Continue to alternate sides, moving with your breath, for a total of 3-5 repetitions on each side.

3. Chair Forward Fold: Sit tall in your chair with your feet flat on the ground and your hands resting on your thighs. Inhale deeply, lengthening your spine. Exhale as you hinge forward from your hips, keeping your back straight and your chest lifted. Bring your hands towards the floor or

rest them on your shins, ankles, or thighs, depending on your flexibility. Hold the forward fold for a few breaths, feeling a gentle stretch in your hamstrings and lower back. Inhale to slowly rise back up to a seated position.

4. Seated Spinal Twist: Sit tall in your chair with your feet flat on the ground and your hands resting on your thighs. Inhale to lengthen your spine, and then exhale as you twist to the right, placing your left hand on the outside of your right thigh and your right hand on the back of the chair for support. Inhale to lengthen the spine once more, and then exhale to deepen the twist, gently looking over your right shoulder. Hold the twist for a few breaths, feeling a gentle stretch along the spine. Inhale to return to center, and then repeat on the other side.

5. Chair Mountain Pose: Sit tall in your chair with your feet flat on the ground and your hands resting on your thighs. Inhale as you reach your arms overhead, palms facing each other. Imagine yourself growing taller as you lengthen through your spine and lift your chest towards the ceiling (Chair Mountain Pose). Hold the pose for a few breaths, feeling a sense of strength and stability in your body. Exhale to release your arms back down to your sides.

6. Seated Sun Salutation: Sit tall in your chair with your feet flat on the ground and your hands resting on your thighs. Inhale as you sweep your arms overhead, reaching up towards the sky. Exhale as you hinge forward from your hips, bringing your hands towards the floor or resting them on your shins, ankles, or thighs (Chair Forward Fold). Inhale to lengthen your spine, and then exhale as you step your right foot back into a lunge position, bringing your hands to the sides of your left foot (Low Lunge). Inhale as you lift your chest and gaze forward. Exhale as

you step your left foot back to meet your right, coming into a plank position. Hold the plank for a breath or two, engaging your core muscles. Inhale to shift your weight forward, coming onto the balls of your feet, and then exhale as you lower your knees, chest, and chin to the floor (Modified Chaturanga). Inhale as you slide forward into a gentle backbend, lifting your chest and gazing up towards the ceiling (Modified Cobra Pose). Exhale as you press back into a Child's Pose, resting your hips on your heels and reaching your arms forward on the floor (Balasana). Take a few breaths in Child's Pose, allowing your body to relax and release any tension. Inhale as you slowly roll up to a seated position, returning to the starting position.

7. Closing Breath: Sit comfortably in your chair with your feet flat on the ground and your hands resting on your thighs. Close your eyes and take a few deep breaths, inhaling through your nose and exhaling through your mouth. With each exhale, imagine releasing any remaining tension or stress from your body and mind. Take a moment to express gratitude for your practice and set an intention for the day ahead. When you're ready, gently open your eyes and return to your day feeling energized and centered.

8. Chair Warrior II Pose (Seated Virabhadrasana II): Sit tall in your chair with your feet flat on the ground and your hands resting on your thighs. Inhale as you extend your right leg out to the side, keeping your foot flat on the ground and your knee bent at a 90-degree angle. Exhale as you extend your arms out to the sides at shoulder height, palms facing down. Gaze over your right fingertips, engaging your core muscles and lengthening through your spine. Hold the pose for a few breaths, feeling strong and grounded like a warrior. Inhale to return to center, and then repeat on the other side.

9. Seated Sun Salutation Variation: Sit tall in your chair with your feet flat on the ground and your hands resting on your thighs. Inhale as you sweep your arms overhead, reaching up towards the sky. Exhale as you hinge forward from your hips, bringing your hands towards the floor or resting them on your shins, ankles, or thighs (Chair Forward Fold). Inhale to lengthen your spine, and then exhale as you step your right foot back into a lunge position, bringing your hands to the sides of your left foot (Low Lunge). Inhale as you lift your chest and gaze forward. Exhale as you step your left foot back to meet your right, coming into a plank position. Hold the plank for a breath or two, engaging your core muscles. Inhale to shift your weight forward, coming onto the balls of your feet, and then exhale as you lower your knees, chest, and chin to the floor (Modified Chaturanga). Inhale as you slide forward into a gentle backbend, lifting your chest and gazing up towards the ceiling (Modified Cobra Pose). Exhale as you press back into a Child's Pose, resting your hips on your heels and reaching your arms forward on the floor (Balasana). Take a few breaths in Child's Pose, allowing your body to relax and release any tension. Inhale as you slowly roll up to a seated position, returning to the starting position.

10. Chair High Lunge: Sit tall in your chair with your feet flat on the ground and your hands resting on your thighs. Inhale as you extend your right leg back, keeping your knee bent and your toes on the ground. Exhale as you lift your chest and reach your arms overhead, coming into a high lunge position with your right foot extended back and your left foot planted firmly on the ground. Hold the pose for a few breaths, engaging your core muscles and lengthening through your spine. Inhale to return to center, and then repeat on the other side.

11. Seated Tree Pose: Sit tall in your chair with your feet flat on the ground and your hands resting on your thighs. Inhale as you lift your right foot off the ground and place the sole of your right foot on the inner left thigh, just above the knee (avoid placing the foot directly on the knee joint). Exhale as you press your right foot into your left thigh and your left thigh into your right foot, finding balance and stability in the pose. Bring your hands to your heart center in a prayer position, or extend your arms overhead for an added challenge. Hold the pose for a few breaths, focusing on your balance and grounding through your seated bones. Inhale to release the pose, and then repeat on the other side.

12. Chair Warrior III Pose (Seated Virabhadrasana III): Sit tall in your chair with your feet flat on the ground and your hands resting on your thighs. Inhale as you extend your right leg back, keeping it parallel to the ground and your toes pointing down. Exhale as you hinge forward from your hips, bringing your torso parallel to the ground and reaching your arms forward in line with your ears (Chair Warrior III). Engage your core muscles and lengthen through your spine, finding balance and stability in the pose. Hold the pose for a few breaths, feeling strong and grounded through your standing leg. Inhale to return to center, and then repeat on the other side.

Midday Stress Relief Routine

The "Midday Stress Relief Routine" is a chair yoga sequence designed to alleviate tension, promote relaxation, and boost energy levels during the middle of the day while also supporting weight loss goals. This routine is especially beneficial for individuals who experience stress or fatigue throughout their busy day and are looking for a quick and effective way to recenter and recharge.

1. Seated Deep Breathing: Begin by sitting comfortably in a chair with your feet flat on the ground and your hands resting on your thighs. Close your eyes or soften your gaze. Take a few moments to focus on your breath, inhaling deeply through your nose and exhaling slowly through your mouth. Allow your breath to become smooth and steady, filling your lungs with air and releasing any tension or stress with each exhale. Continue this deep breathing for several rounds, allowing it to calm your nervous system and center your mind.

2. Neck Rolls: Sit tall in your chair with your feet flat on the ground and your hands resting on your thighs. Inhale deeply and as you exhale, gently lower your chin towards your chest, feeling a stretch along the back of your neck. Inhale and roll your head to the right, bringing your right ear towards your right shoulder. Exhale and roll your head back down towards your chest. Inhale and roll your head to the left, bringing your left ear towards your left shoulder. Exhale and roll your head back down towards your chest. Continue this slow and gentle movement, allowing your breath to guide the motion of your head. Repeat for several rounds, feeling any tension or tightness in your neck gradually release.

3. Seated Forward Fold: Sit tall in your chair with your feet flat on the ground and your hands resting on your thighs. Inhale deeply and as you exhale, hinge forward from your hips, bringing your chest towards your thighs and reaching your hands towards the ground. Allow your head to hang heavy and relax your neck. Feel a gentle stretch along your spine and the backs of your legs. Hold this seated forward fold for several breaths, breathing deeply into any areas of tightness or tension. Inhale and slowly return to an upright position.

4. Chair Cat-Cow Stretch: Sit tall in your chair with your feet flat on the ground and your hands resting on your thighs. Inhale deeply and as you exhale, round your spine, tucking your chin towards your chest and drawing your belly button towards your spine. Feel a stretch along your back. Inhale and arch your back, lifting your chest and opening your heart towards the sky. Allow your belly to relax and your shoulders to soften. Continue flowing between these two movements, syncing your breath with the motion of your spine. Repeat for several rounds, allowing your breath to guide the movement and release any tension in your back.

5. Seated Twists: Sit tall in your chair with your feet flat on the ground and your hands resting on your thighs. Inhale deeply and as you exhale, twist your torso to the right, placing your left hand on the outside of your right thigh and your right hand on the back of your chair. Gently gaze over your right shoulder, feeling a stretch along your spine and the sides of your torso. Hold this seated twist for several breaths, breathing deeply into the twist and feeling any tension in your back release. Inhale and return to center, then exhale and twist to the left, repeating the stretch on the opposite side. Hold for several breaths, allowing the twist to deepen with each exhale. Inhale and return to center.

6. Seated Side Stretches: Sit tall in your chair with your feet flat on the ground and your hands resting on your thighs. Inhale deeply and as you exhale, reach your right arm up towards the sky, stretching it overhead and leaning gently to the left. Feel a stretch along the right side of your body. Hold this seated side stretch for several breaths, breathing deeply into the stretch and feeling any tension in your side release. Inhale and return to center, then exhale and repeat the

stretch on the opposite side, reaching your left arm up towards the sky and leaning gently to the right. Hold for several breaths, allowing the stretch to deepen with each exhale. Inhale and return to center.

7. Seated Spinal Twist: Sit tall in your chair with your feet flat on the ground and your hands resting on your thighs. Inhale deeply and as you exhale, twist your torso to the right, placing your left hand on the outside of your right thigh and your right hand on the back of your chair. Gently gaze over your right shoulder, feeling a stretch along your spine and the sides of your torso. Hold this seated twist for several breaths, breathing deeply into the twist and feeling any tension in your back release. Inhale and return to center, then exhale and twist to the left, repeating the stretch on the opposite side. Hold for several breaths, allowing the twist to deepen with each exhale. Inhale and return to center.

8. Seated Mountain Pose: Sit tall in your chair with your feet flat on the ground and your hands resting on your thighs. Close your eyes or soften your gaze. Take a few moments to focus on your posture, lengthening your spine and lifting your chest towards the sky. Allow your shoulders to relax away from your ears and your hands to rest comfortably on your thighs. Take a few deep breaths in this seated mountain pose, feeling grounded and centered in your body. Allow any remaining tension or stress to melt away with each exhale.

9. Seated Eagle Arms: Sit tall in your chair with your feet flat on the ground and your hands resting on your thighs. Inhale deeply and as you exhale, cross your right arm under your left arm, bringing your palms together if possible. Lift your elbows slightly and draw your shoulder blades

down your back. Hold this seated eagle arms pose for several breaths, feeling a stretch between your shoulder blades and along your upper back. Inhale and release, then repeat on the opposite side, crossing your left arm under your right arm.

10. Seated Forward Bend with Twist: Sit tall in your chair with your feet flat on the ground and your hands resting on your thighs. Inhale deeply and as you exhale, hinge forward from your hips, bringing your chest towards your thighs. Allow your hands to reach towards the ground or grab hold of the sides of your chair for support. Inhale and lengthen your spine, then exhale and twist your torso to the right, placing your left hand on the outside of your right thigh and your right hand on the back of your chair. Gently gaze over your right shoulder. Hold this seated forward bend with twist for several breaths, feeling a stretch along your spine and the sides of your torso. Inhale and return to center, then exhale and repeat the twist on the opposite side.

11. Seated Leg Extension with Forward Fold: Sit tall in your chair with your feet flat on the ground and your hands resting on your thighs. Inhale deeply and as you exhale, extend your right leg forward, flexing your foot. Keep your left foot planted on the ground for support. Inhale and lengthen your spine, then exhale and hinge forward from your hips, bringing your chest towards your thigh. Allow your hands to reach towards your right foot or grab hold of the sides of your chair for support. Hold this seated leg extension with forward fold for several breaths, feeling a stretch along the back of your right leg. Inhale and return to an upright position, then exhale and repeat on the opposite side.

12. Seated Sun Salutation: Sit tall in your chair with your feet flat on the ground and your hands resting on your thighs. Inhale and sweep your arms overhead, reaching towards the sky. Exhale and bring your hands down to heart center, pressing your palms together. Inhale and reach your arms overhead again, lengthening your spine. Exhale and hinge forward from your hips, bringing your chest towards your thighs. Inhale and lengthen your spine, then exhale and twist your torso to the right, placing your left hand on the outside of your right thigh and your right hand on the back of your chair. Gently gaze over your right shoulder. Inhale and return to center, then exhale and repeat the twist on the opposite side. Inhale and return to center, then exhale and sweep your arms down to your sides. Repeat this seated sun salutation for several rounds, flowing with your breath and allowing each movement to be smooth and fluid.

13. Seated Warrior II: Sit tall in your chair with your feet flat on the ground and your hands resting on your thighs. Inhale and extend your right leg out to the side, keeping your foot flat on the ground. Exhale and bend your right knee, bringing it in line with your right ankle. Inhale and extend your arms out to the sides, reaching through your fingertips. Gaze over your right fingertips, feeling strong and grounded in your seated warrior II pose. Hold for several breaths, then inhale and straighten your right leg, returning to center. Repeat on the opposite side, extending your left leg out to the side and bending your left knee. Inhale and extend your arms out to the sides, reaching through your fingertips. Gaze over your left fingertips, feeling strong and grounded in your seated warrior II pose. Hold for several breaths, then inhale and return to center.

14. Seated Tree Pose: Sit tall in your chair with your feet flat on the ground and your hands resting on your thighs. Inhale and lift your right foot off the ground, bringing the sole of your foot to rest on your left inner thigh or calf. Exhale and press your right foot into your inner thigh or calf, finding balance in your seated tree pose. Inhale and reach your arms overhead, lengthening your spine. Exhale and bring your hands down to heart center, pressing your palms together. Hold this seated tree pose for several breaths, feeling grounded and stable. Inhale and return your foot to the ground, then exhale and repeat on the opposite side, lifting your left foot off the ground and bringing the sole of your foot to rest on your right inner thigh or calf.

15. Seated Meditation: Sit tall in your chair with your feet flat on the ground and your hands resting on your thighs. Close your eyes or soften your gaze. Take a few moments to focus on your breath, inhaling deeply through your nose and exhaling slowly through your mouth. Allow your breath to become smooth and steady, grounding you in the present.

Evening Relaxation Routine

The "Evening Relaxation Routine" is a soothing chair yoga sequence designed to promote relaxation and stress relief, making it an excellent choice for winding down at the end of the day while also supporting weight loss efforts by reducing cortisol levels and promoting better sleep quality. This gentle routine focuses on stretching and releasing tension in the body, calming the mind, and preparing for restorative sleep. Here's a sample chair yoga routine:

1. Seated Mountain Pose (Tadasana): Sit comfortably in your chair with your feet flat on the ground and your spine tall. Rest your hands on your thighs, palms facing down. Close your eyes and take a few deep breaths, grounding yourself and bringing awareness to your body.

2. Seated Side Stretch: Inhale as you reach your arms overhead, interlacing your fingers and pressing your palms towards the ceiling. Exhale and gently lean to the right, stretching the left side of your body. Hold for a few breaths, feeling the stretch along your left side. Inhale to come back to center, and exhale as you lean to the left, stretching the right side of your body. Hold for a few breaths, then return to center.

3. Seated Cat-Cow Stretch: Place your hands on your knees. Inhale as you arch your back, lifting your chest and tilting your pelvis forward (Cow Pose). Exhale as you round your spine, tucking your chin to your chest and tilting your pelvis backward (Cat Pose). Repeat this flowing movement, synchronizing your breath with the movement of your spine.

4. Seated Forward Fold: Inhale as you lengthen your spine, and exhale as you hinge forward from your hips, keeping your back straight. Fold forward as far as comfortable, allowing your chest to rest on your thighs and your arms to hang towards the floor. Hold for a few breaths, feeling the stretch in your lower back and hamstrings. Inhale to slowly roll back up to a seated position.

5. Seated Spinal Twist: Sit tall in your chair with your feet flat on the ground. Inhale as you lengthen your spine, and exhale as you twist to the right, placing your left hand on the outside of

your right thigh and your right hand on the back of the chair. Hold the twist for a few breaths, feeling the gentle stretch in your spine and torso. Inhale to come back to center, and exhale as you twist to the left, repeating the stretch on the opposite side.

6. Seated Relaxation: Sit comfortably in your chair with your feet flat on the ground and your hands resting on your thighs. Close your eyes and take several deep breaths, allowing your body to relax and release any remaining tension. Focus on softening your muscles and letting go of any thoughts or worries. Stay in this seated relaxation pose for several minutes, allowing yourself to fully unwind and prepare for restful sleep.

7. Closing Meditation: With your eyes still closed, bring your hands together at your heart center in a prayer position (Anjali Mudra). Take a moment to express gratitude for the practice and for the opportunity to nourish your body and mind. Set an intention for restful sleep and overall well-being. Take one final deep breath in and exhale fully, releasing any tension or stress. When you're ready, gently open your eyes and return to the present moment.

8. Seated Forward Bend with Shoulder Opener: Sit at the edge of your chair with your feet flat on the ground. Interlace your fingers behind your back and straighten your arms, allowing your shoulders to gently roll back. Inhale as you lengthen your spine, and exhale as you fold forward from your hips, bringing your chest towards your thighs. Let your arms fall forward overhead, allowing gravity to deepen the stretch in your shoulders and upper back. Hold for a few breaths, feeling a gentle release of tension in your upper body.

9. Seated Eagle Arms: Sit comfortably in your chair with your feet flat on the ground. Extend your arms straight out in front of you at shoulder height. Cross your right arm over your left arm, bringing your palms together in front of your face. Bend your elbows and bring your forearms perpendicular to the ground, wrapping your right forearm around your left forearm. Lift your elbows slightly and press your palms together. Hold this seated eagle arms pose for a few breaths, feeling a stretch in your shoulders and upper back. Repeat on the other side, crossing your left arm over your right arm.

10. Seated Neck Release: Sit tall in your chair with your feet flat on the ground. Inhale as you lengthen your spine, and exhale as you gently drop your right ear towards your right shoulder, feeling a stretch along the left side of your neck. Hold for a few breaths, then inhale to come back to center. Exhale as you drop your left ear towards your left shoulder, feeling a stretch along the right side of your neck. Hold for a few breaths, then return to center. Repeat this seated neck release on both sides, moving slowly and mindfully.

11. Seated Forward Bend with Twist: Sit at the edge of your chair with your feet flat on the ground. Inhale as you lengthen your spine, and exhale as you fold forward from your hips, bringing your chest towards your thighs. Place your right hand on the outside of your left knee and your left hand on the back of the chair. Inhale to lengthen your spine, and exhale as you gently twist to the left, looking over your left shoulder. Hold for a few breaths, feeling a stretch in your spine and torso. Inhale to come back to center, and repeat on the other side, twisting to the right.

12. Seated Meditation: After completing the chair yoga poses, come to a comfortable seated position in your chair with your feet flat on the ground and your hands resting on your thighs. Close your eyes and take several deep breaths, allowing your body and mind to relax completely. Focus on your breath, observing the natural rhythm of inhalation and exhalation. If your mind wanders, gently bring your attention back to your breath. Stay in this seated meditation for several minutes, allowing yourself to experience a sense of inner peace and calm.

<u>**Chapter 5: Incorporating Mindfulness and Meditation**</u>

<u>**Benefits of Mindfulness and Meditation**</u>

Mindfulness and meditation offer a wide range of benefits that positively impact various aspects of our physical, mental, and emotional well-being. Here are some key benefits:

1. Stress Reduction: Mindfulness and meditation techniques help reduce the body's stress response by activating the relaxation response. Regular practice lowers levels of cortisol, the stress hormone, leading to a decrease in overall stress levels and an increased sense of calm and relaxation.

2. Improved Emotional Regulation: Mindfulness and meditation cultivate awareness of thoughts, emotions, and bodily sensations without judgment. This enhanced self-awareness enables individuals to respond to challenging situations with greater emotional resilience, leading to improved mood regulation and decreased reactivity.

3. Enhanced Focus and Concentration: Mindfulness practices involve training the mind to stay focused on the present moment. Regular meditation strengthens the brain's attentional circuits, improving concentration, cognitive function, and the ability to sustain attention on tasks.

4. Better Sleep Quality: Mindfulness and meditation promote relaxation and reduce rumination, leading to improved sleep quality and duration. Individuals who practice mindfulness techniques report experiencing fewer sleep disturbances and better overall sleep patterns.

5. Pain Management: Mindfulness-based interventions have been shown to effectively reduce the perception of pain and improve pain tolerance. By cultivating non-judgmental awareness of physical sensations, individuals can develop a healthier relationship with pain and learn to cope with it more effectively.

6. Enhanced Self-Awareness and Acceptance: Mindfulness and meditation encourage self-reflection and introspection, leading to a deeper understanding of oneself and one's values. This increased self-awareness fosters self-acceptance, compassion, and a greater sense of overall well-being.

7. Reduced Symptoms of Anxiety and Depression: Mindfulness-based interventions have been found to significantly reduce symptoms of anxiety and depression. By teaching individuals to observe their thoughts and emotions without attachment or judgment, mindfulness practices help break the cycle of negative thinking patterns associated with these mental health conditions.

8. Improved Relationships: Mindfulness and meditation cultivate qualities such as empathy, compassion, and non-reactivity, which are essential for healthy interpersonal relationships. By fostering a deeper understanding of oneself and others, mindfulness practices promote more authentic and meaningful connections with others.

9. Enhanced Resilience: Regular mindfulness and meditation practice build psychological resilience, enabling individuals to bounce back more effectively from life's challenges and

setbacks. By developing a greater capacity to cope with stress and adversity, individuals can experience greater overall resilience and well-being.

10. Greater Sense of Purpose and Meaning: Mindfulness and meditation practices encourage individuals to connect with their inner values and aspirations, leading to a deeper sense of purpose and meaning in life. By fostering a greater alignment between one's actions and values, mindfulness cultivates a more fulfilling and purpose-driven life.

11. Enhanced Cognitive Function: Mindfulness and meditation practices have been linked to improvements in cognitive function, including memory, attention, and executive function. By training the brain to focus on the present moment and maintain sustained attention, these practices strengthen neural networks associated with cognitive processing, leading to better overall cognitive performance.

12. Increased Emotional Intelligence: Mindfulness and meditation cultivate emotional intelligence by fostering greater self-awareness, self-regulation, and empathy. Individuals who practice mindfulness techniques develop a deeper understanding of their own emotions and learn to respond to them in a more adaptive manner. Additionally, they become more attuned to the emotions of others, leading to improved interpersonal relationships and communication skills.

13. Enhanced Creativity: Mindfulness and meditation practices promote divergent thinking, which is crucial for creativity and problem-solving. By quieting the mind and reducing cognitive

rigidity, these practices create space for innovative ideas to emerge. Regular meditation has been shown to enhance creative thinking abilities and inspire new perspectives and insights.

14. Improved Physical Health: Mindfulness and meditation have been associated with numerous physical health benefits, including reduced blood pressure, improved cardiovascular health, and enhanced immune function. By reducing stress and inflammation in the body, these practices support overall physical well-being and resilience.

15. Pregnancy and Childbirth: Mindfulness-based interventions have been shown to be beneficial during pregnancy and childbirth, helping expectant mothers manage stress, anxiety, and pain during labor. Mindfulness techniques, such as focused breathing and body scanning, can promote relaxation and facilitate a more positive childbirth experience.

16. Substance Abuse Recovery: Mindfulness-based interventions have been used as an adjunctive treatment for individuals recovering from substance abuse disorders. These practices help individuals develop greater awareness of their cravings, triggers, and habitual patterns, empowering them to make healthier choices and maintain sobriety.

17. Post-Traumatic Growth: Mindfulness and meditation have been shown to facilitate post-traumatic growth, the process of positive psychological change that occurs in the aftermath of adversity. By cultivating acceptance, resilience, and a sense of meaning, these practices support individuals in finding strength and personal growth in the face of trauma and adversity.

18. Spiritual Growth: For many individuals, mindfulness and meditation serve as pathways to spiritual growth and self-transcendence. These practices facilitate a deeper connection with oneself, others, and the world, leading to a greater sense of interconnectedness and spiritual fulfillment.

19. Workplace Benefits: Mindfulness-based interventions have been increasingly implemented in workplace settings to promote employee well-being, productivity, and job satisfaction. These practices help employees manage stress, improve focus and concentration, and enhance interpersonal relationships, ultimately creating a more positive and supportive work environment.

20. Lifelong Learning: Mindfulness and meditation encourage a growth mindset and a willingness to embrace lifelong learning and personal growth. By fostering curiosity, openness, and a non-judgmental attitude, these practices support continuous self-improvement and intellectual curiosity throughout life.

Chair Yoga Meditation Techniques

Chair yoga meditation techniques offer a gentle and accessible way to cultivate mindfulness, relaxation, and inner peace while seated comfortably in a chair. These techniques can be adapted to suit individuals of all ages and physical abilities, making them ideal for those who may have difficulty practicing traditional seated meditation on the floor. Here are some chair yoga meditation techniques to explore:

1. Breath Awareness: Sit comfortably in your chair with your feet flat on the ground and your hands resting on your thighs. Close your eyes or soften your gaze. Bring your attention to your breath, noticing the sensation of the breath as it enters and leaves your body. Observe the natural rhythm of your breath without trying to control it. If your mind wanders, gently guide your attention back to your breath. Practice this breath awareness meditation for several minutes, allowing yourself to become fully present in the moment.

2. Body Scan: Sit comfortably in your chair with your feet flat on the ground and your hands resting on your thighs. Close your eyes or soften your gaze. Begin by bringing your awareness to your feet, noticing any sensations of warmth, tingling, or pressure. Slowly move your attention upward through your body, scanning each area from your feet to the top of your head. Notice any areas of tension or discomfort, and imagine sending your breath to those areas to help release any tension or tightness. Practice this body scan meditation, allowing yourself to relax deeply into the present moment.

3. Mindful Movement: Incorporate gentle movements into your chair yoga practice to cultivate mindfulness and presence. As you inhale, lift your arms overhead, and as you exhale, lower them back down to your sides. Coordinate your breath with your movements, allowing your breath to guide the pace of your movements. Notice the sensation of the air moving through your body as you breathe and move. This mindful movement meditation helps to synchronize breath and movement, promoting relaxation and awareness.

4. Visualization: Sit comfortably in your chair with your feet flat on the ground and your hands resting on your thighs. Close your eyes or soften your gaze. Visualize a peaceful scene, such as a calm lake, a serene forest, or a tranquil beach. Imagine yourself fully immersed in this scene, noticing the sights, sounds, and sensations around you. Allow yourself to relax deeply into this visualization, letting go of any tension or stress. Practice this visualization meditation for several minutes, allowing yourself to experience a sense of inner peace and tranquility.

5. Loving-Kindness (Metta) Meditation: Sit comfortably in your chair with your feet flat on the ground and your hands resting on your thighs. Close your eyes or soften your gaze. Begin by directing loving-kindness towards yourself, silently repeating phrases such as "May I be happy, may I be healthy, may I be safe, may I live with ease." Then, extend this loving-kindness outward to others, silently repeating similar phrases for loved ones, acquaintances, and even difficult individuals. Practice this loving-kindness meditation, allowing yourself to cultivate feelings of compassion, empathy, and goodwill towards yourself and others.

6. Mantra Meditation: Sit comfortably in your chair with your feet flat on the ground and your hands resting on your thighs. Close your eyes or soften your gaze. Choose a simple, soothing mantra or phrase to repeat silently to yourself with each breath. This could be a word like "peace," "love," or "serenity," or a phrase like "I am calm and centered." As you inhale, silently repeat the first half of the mantra, and as you exhale, silently repeat the second half. Allow the repetition of the mantra to anchor your mind and deepen your sense of relaxation and presence.

7. Sound Meditation: Sit comfortably in your chair with your feet flat on the ground and your hands resting on your thighs. Close your eyes or soften your gaze. Bring your awareness to the sounds around you, both near and far. Notice the sounds of traffic, birdsong, or the hum of appliances. Instead of labeling or judging the sounds, simply observe them with curiosity and openness. Allow the sounds to come and go, like waves washing over you. This sound meditation can help cultivate a sense of spacious awareness and presence.

8. Gratitude Meditation: Sit comfortably in your chair with your feet flat on the ground and your hands resting on your thighs. Close your eyes or soften your gaze. Take a few moments to reflect on the things you are grateful for in your life. These could be simple things like a warm cup of tea, a kind smile from a friend, or the beauty of nature. With each breath, silently express gratitude for these blessings in your life. Feel the warmth and appreciation filling your heart with each breath. This gratitude meditation can help shift your focus from what is lacking to what is abundant in your life, fostering a sense of contentment and well-being.

9. Body Awareness Meditation: Sit comfortably in your chair with your feet flat on the ground and your hands resting on your thighs. Close your eyes or soften your gaze. Bring your awareness to different parts of your body, starting from your feet and moving upward to your head. Notice any sensations, tension, or areas of tightness in each part of your body. With each breath, imagine sending a wave of relaxation and healing energy to that area, allowing it to soften and release any tension. This body awareness meditation can help you connect with your body and cultivate a sense of ease and relaxation.

10. Breath Counting Meditation: Sit comfortably in your chair with your feet flat on the ground and your hands resting on your thighs. Close your eyes or soften your gaze. Begin by taking a few deep breaths to settle into your body. Then, start counting your breaths silently in your mind, starting from one and counting up to ten. With each inhale and exhale, count one number higher until you reach ten, and then start again at one. If you lose track or your mind wanders, simply return to counting your breaths from one. This breath counting meditation can help anchor your attention and calm your mind.

Chapter 6: Nutrition Tips for Weight Loss

Importance of Nutrition in Weight Loss

Nutrition plays a pivotal role in weight loss, as it directly impacts the body's energy balance and metabolism. Here are several key reasons highlighting the importance of nutrition in weight loss:

1. Caloric Balance: Weight loss ultimately comes down to achieving a negative energy balance, where the calories consumed are fewer than the calories expended. This creates a caloric deficit, prompting the body to use stored energy (in the form of fat) to meet its energy needs, thus leading to weight loss. Proper nutrition helps individuals maintain this caloric balance by providing essential nutrients while controlling calorie intake.

2. Nutrient Density: Choosing nutrient-dense foods—those that are rich in vitamins, minerals, and other essential nutrients—helps ensure that the body receives the necessary fuel for optimal functioning while consuming fewer calories. Nutrient-dense foods include fruits, vegetables, whole grains, lean proteins, and healthy fats, which provide satiety and promote overall health while supporting weight loss.

3. Metabolic Health: Proper nutrition supports metabolic health by regulating blood sugar levels, optimizing insulin sensitivity, and promoting efficient energy metabolism. A diet rich in whole, unprocessed foods helps stabilize blood sugar levels, preventing spikes and crashes that can lead to increased hunger and overeating, ultimately supporting weight loss efforts.

4. Muscle Preservation: During weight loss, it's essential to preserve lean muscle mass while reducing body fat. Adequate protein intake, along with resistance training exercise, helps support muscle maintenance and growth, which is crucial for maintaining metabolic rate and overall physical function. Proper nutrition provides the amino acids necessary for muscle repair and growth, ensuring that weight loss consists primarily of fat rather than muscle tissue.

5. Hormonal Balance: Nutrition plays a significant role in hormonal balance, which influences appetite regulation, metabolism, and fat storage. Consuming a balanced diet that includes a variety of macronutrients—such as carbohydrates, proteins, and fats—in appropriate proportions helps regulate hormones like leptin, ghrelin, insulin, and cortisol, which play key roles in hunger, satiety, and fat metabolism.

6. Satiety and Hunger Management: Proper nutrition supports feelings of satiety and helps manage hunger, which are essential factors in maintaining a calorie deficit for weight loss. Foods high in fiber, protein, and healthy fats promote feelings of fullness and satisfaction, reducing the likelihood of overeating or succumbing to cravings, ultimately supporting weight loss efforts.

7. Long-Term Health and Sustainability: Optimal nutrition not only supports short-term weight loss goals but also contributes to long-term health and weight maintenance. A balanced diet rich in whole, nutrient-dense foods provides essential vitamins, minerals, and antioxidants that support overall health and well-being, reducing the risk of chronic diseases and promoting longevity.

8. Energy Levels and Performance: Nutrition plays a crucial role in providing the energy needed for physical activity and exercise, which is an essential component of any weight loss plan. Adequate intake of carbohydrates, fats, and proteins ensures sustained energy levels, optimizing performance during workouts and daily activities. Proper nutrition also supports recovery and muscle repair post-exercise, enhancing overall fitness and metabolic efficiency.

9. Metabolic Adaptation: The body's metabolism can adapt to changes in calorie intake and composition, affecting weight loss progress. A well-balanced diet that includes adequate protein, healthy fats, and complex carbohydrates helps prevent metabolic adaptation and supports a more sustainable rate of weight loss over time. This approach promotes metabolic flexibility, enabling the body to efficiently utilize stored fat for energy while preserving lean muscle mass.

10. Behavioral and Psychological Factors: Nutrition impacts various behavioral and psychological factors that influence food choices, eating behaviors, and adherence to weight loss strategies. Nutrient-dense foods rich in fiber, vitamins, and minerals promote feelings of satisfaction and well-being, reducing the likelihood of emotional eating or cravings for unhealthy foods. Additionally, adopting a balanced and sustainable approach to nutrition fosters a positive relationship with food and supports long-term adherence to healthy eating habits.

11. Gut Health: Emerging research suggests that gut health plays a significant role in weight management and overall health. A balanced diet that includes fiber-rich foods, probiotics, and prebiotics supports a diverse and healthy gut microbiome, which is associated with improved

digestion, nutrient absorption, and metabolism. Maintaining gut health through proper nutrition may contribute to more efficient weight loss and long-term weight management.

12. Nutrition Quality vs. Quantity: While calorie intake is a crucial factor in weight loss, the quality of those calories also matters. Consuming nutrient-dense foods provides essential vitamins, minerals, and antioxidants that support overall health and well-being, beyond just weight loss. Prioritizing whole, minimally processed foods over highly processed, calorie-dense foods helps optimize nutrition quality, supporting both weight loss and long-term health goals.

13. Individualized Approach: It's essential to recognize that nutrition needs vary among individuals based on factors such as age, gender, activity level, metabolic rate, and underlying health conditions. An individualized approach to nutrition considers these factors and tailors dietary recommendations to meet specific needs and goals. Consulting with a registered dietitian or nutritionist can provide personalized guidance and support for effective weight loss strategies.

14. Education and Empowerment: Embracing a holistic approach to nutrition empowers individuals to make informed food choices and take control of their health and weight loss journey. Education about the nutritional value of foods, portion sizes, meal planning, and cooking skills equips individuals with the knowledge and tools needed to navigate food environments and make healthier choices that support their weight loss goals.

Healthy Eating Tips for Seniors Over 60

Maintaining a healthy diet is crucial for seniors over 60 to support overall health, vitality, and quality of life. As individuals age, their nutritional needs may change, making it essential to prioritize nutrient-dense foods that support optimal health and well-being. Here are some healthy eating tips tailored specifically for seniors over 60:

1. Focus on Nutrient-Dense Foods: Choose foods that are rich in essential nutrients such as vitamins, minerals, fiber, and antioxidants. Include a variety of fruits, vegetables, whole grains, lean proteins, and healthy fats in your diet to ensure you're getting a wide range of nutrients to support overall health.

2. Prioritize Protein: Protein is essential for maintaining muscle mass, supporting immune function, and promoting overall health in seniors. Include sources of lean protein in your diet such as poultry, fish, beans, lentils, tofu, eggs, and dairy products. Aim to include protein with each meal to support muscle health and satiety.

3. Stay Hydrated: Dehydration is common among seniors and can lead to various health issues such as urinary tract infections, constipation, and cognitive decline. Make sure to drink plenty of fluids throughout the day, including water, herbal teas, and low-sugar beverages, to stay properly hydrated.

4. Mindful Portion Control: As metabolism tends to slow down with age, it's essential to be mindful of portion sizes to prevent overeating and maintain a healthy weight. Use smaller plates and bowls, and pay attention to hunger and fullness cues to avoid overeating.

5. Include Fiber-Rich Foods: Fiber is essential for digestive health, heart health, and weight management. Include plenty of fiber-rich foods in your diet such as fruits, vegetables, whole grains, legumes, nuts, and seeds to support digestive regularity and overall health.

6. Limit Processed Foods: Minimize your intake of processed and packaged foods that are high in added sugars, unhealthy fats, and sodium. Instead, opt for whole, minimally processed foods that are nutrient-dense and support overall health.

7. Practice Mindful Eating: Pay attention to your body's hunger and fullness cues, and practice mindful eating by savoring each bite and enjoying the flavors and textures of your food. Eating slowly and mindfully can help prevent overeating and promote greater satisfaction from meals.

8. Choose Healthy Fats: Include sources of healthy fats in your diet such as avocados, nuts, seeds, olive oil, and fatty fish like salmon and mackerel. These fats provide essential fatty acids that support heart health, brain function, and overall well-being.

9. Be Flexible and Enjoy Moderation: While it's essential to prioritize nutrient-dense foods, it's also important to enjoy your favorite foods in moderation. Allow yourself occasional treats and indulgences while maintaining balance and moderation in your overall diet.

10. Consult with a Registered Dietitian: If you have specific dietary concerns or health conditions, consider consulting with a registered dietitian who can provide personalized nutrition guidance tailored to your individual needs and goals.

11. Vitamin and Mineral Supplementation: While it's ideal to obtain nutrients from whole foods, some seniors may have difficulty meeting their nutritional needs through diet alone. Consider taking a multivitamin or specific supplements as recommended by your healthcare provider to fill any gaps in your diet, particularly for nutrients like vitamin B12, vitamin D, calcium, and magnesium, which may be more challenging to obtain from food as you age.

12. Mind Your Sodium Intake: Seniors are often more sensitive to the effects of sodium, which can contribute to high blood pressure and other cardiovascular issues. To help manage blood pressure and overall heart health, limit your intake of high-sodium foods such as processed meats, canned soups, and salty snacks. Instead, flavor your meals with herbs, spices, and citrus juices to enhance taste without relying on excessive salt.

13. Consider Texture Modifications: Some seniors may experience dental issues, swallowing difficulties, or changes in taste and texture perception as they age, making certain foods more challenging to eat. If you have difficulty chewing or swallowing, consider incorporating softer, more easily digestible foods into your diet, such as steamed vegetables, smoothies, soups, and pureed dishes. Additionally, be mindful of foods that may cause discomfort or irritation, such as spicy or acidic foods.

14. Meal Planning and Preparation: Planning and preparing meals in advance can help ensure you have nutritious options readily available and reduce reliance on convenience or fast foods. Consider batch cooking and freezing portions for later use, using slow cookers or Instant Pots for easy meal preparation, or exploring meal delivery services that offer healthy, senior-friendly options.

15. Stay Social and Engaged: Eating is not just about nourishment; it's also a social and enjoyable activity. Share meals with friends, family, or participate in community meal programs to stay connected and engaged. Socializing during meals can enhance appetite, promote mindful eating, and contribute to overall well-being.

16. Be Mindful of Medication Interactions: Some medications can interact with certain foods, nutrients, or dietary supplements, potentially affecting their effectiveness or causing adverse effects. If you're taking medications, consult with your healthcare provider or pharmacist to ensure there are no contraindications with specific foods or supplements in your diet.

17. Monitor Fluid Intake: In addition to staying hydrated with water, consider incorporating hydrating foods with high water content into your diet, such as fruits (e.g., watermelon, oranges), vegetables (e.g., cucumbers, celery), soups, and herbal teas. Monitor your fluid intake, particularly if you have conditions like heart failure or kidney disease that may require fluid restriction, and consult with your healthcare provider for personalized recommendations.

18. Listen to Your Body: Pay attention to how different foods make you feel and adjust your diet accordingly. If certain foods cause digestive discomfort, bloating, or other adverse reactions, consider eliminating or reducing them from your diet. Experiment with different foods and eating patterns to find what works best for your body and overall well-being.

19. Stay Informed and Seek Support: Stay informed about nutrition and healthy eating guidelines for seniors, and don't hesitate to seek support from healthcare professionals, registered dietitians, or nutritionists if you have questions or concerns about your diet. They can provide personalized guidance and support to help you make informed choices that promote optimal health and well-being.

<u>**Chapter 7: Overcoming Challenges and Staying Motivated**</u>

<u>**Dealing with Physical Limitations**</u>

Dealing with physical limitations as a senior during chair yoga for weight loss involves modifying poses to suit your abilities. Focus on gentle movements that still engage your muscles, such as seated twists or arm stretches. Utilize props like blocks or straps to assist in achieving poses comfortably. Listen to your body, taking breaks when needed, and gradually increase intensity over time.

Let's dive deeper into how seniors can effectively manage physical limitations while practicing chair yoga for weight loss:

1. Start Slowly: Begin with basic chair yoga poses and gradually progress to more challenging ones as your strength and flexibility improve. Don't push yourself too hard initially; listen to your body's cues and only do what feels comfortable.

2. Focus on Range of Motion: Chair yoga can help improve flexibility and range of motion, which is particularly beneficial for seniors with physical limitations. Focus on gentle stretches that target different muscle groups, such as shoulder rolls, neck stretches, and seated forward bends.

3. Use Props: Props like blocks, straps, and pillows can provide support and stability during chair yoga poses. For example, using a pillow behind your back can provide extra support during seated poses, while a strap can help you extend your reach during stretches.

4. Modify Poses: Don't be afraid to modify poses to suit your individual needs and limitations. For example, if you have limited mobility in your legs, you can perform seated versions of standing poses like Warrior I or Tree Pose. Your yoga instructor can provide guidance on how to modify poses effectively.

5. Focus on Breathing: Pay attention to your breath during chair yoga practice. Deep, mindful breathing can help reduce stress, improve concentration, and enhance relaxation. Incorporate breathing exercises like deep belly breathing or alternate nostril breathing into your practice.

6. Listen to Your Body: It's essential to listen to your body and respect its limitations. If a pose feels uncomfortable or causes pain, ease out of it immediately and try a modified version or a different pose. Remember, yoga is about honoring your body and its unique needs.

7. Stay Consistent: Consistency is key when it comes to seeing results from chair yoga for weight loss. Aim to practice regularly, even if it's just for a few minutes each day. Consistent practice can help improve strength, flexibility, and overall well-being over time.

Setting Realistic Goals

Setting realistic goals as a senior practicing chair yoga for weight loss is crucial for progress and motivation. Here's how you can establish achievable goals:

1. Assess Your Current Fitness Level: Begin by assessing your current fitness level and understanding your physical limitations. Consider factors such as mobility, flexibility, strength, and endurance. This assessment will help you set realistic goals that are tailored to your abilities.

2. Consult with a Healthcare Professional: Before setting any fitness goals, consult with your healthcare provider or a qualified fitness professional. They can provide valuable insights into your health status, offer recommendations, and help you set realistic goals that align with your overall well-being.

3. Identify Specific Objectives: Instead of setting broad goals like "lose weight," identify specific objectives related to chair yoga practice. For example, your goals could include improving flexibility, increasing muscle strength, enhancing balance and stability, or reducing stress levels.

4. Use the SMART Criteria: Apply the SMART criteria to your goal-setting process. Ensure that your goals are Specific, Measurable, Achievable, Relevant, and Time-bound. For instance, instead of setting a vague goal like "improve flexibility," a SMART goal could be "increase hamstring flexibility by 1 inch within three months."

5. Break Down Goals into Smaller Steps: Break down larger goals into smaller, manageable steps or milestones. This approach makes goals less overwhelming and allows you to track progress more effectively. Celebrate each small achievement along the way to stay motivated.

6. Consider Non-Scale Victories: While weight loss may be a goal, focus on non-scale victories as well. Celebrate improvements in mobility, balance, strength, flexibility, and overall well-being. These achievements are just as important and can contribute to your overall success.

7. Be Realistic and Flexible: Be realistic about what you can achieve within a given timeframe, considering your age, fitness level, and any physical limitations. Adjust your goals as needed based on your progress and any changes in your health or circumstances.

8. Listen to Your Body: Pay attention to your body's signals and adjust your goals and intensity of practice accordingly. It's essential to prioritize safety and avoid pushing yourself beyond your limits, especially as a senior.

9. Track Your Progress: Keep track of your progress using a journal, fitness app, or other tracking tools. Documenting your achievements, challenges, and improvements can help you stay accountable and motivated throughout your chair yoga journey.

10. Celebrate Achievements: Celebrate your accomplishments, no matter how small. Acknowledge your efforts and progress, and treat yourself with kindness and encouragement along the way.

11. Focus on Functional Fitness: Consider setting goals that enhance your functional fitness, which includes activities necessary for daily living. Examples include improving the ability to

stand up from a chair, reaching overhead to grab items, or maintaining balance while walking. These goals directly impact your quality of life and independence.

12. Emphasize Consistency Over Intensity: As a senior, consistency in your chair yoga practice is key. Rather than aiming for intense workouts, prioritize regularity in your practice sessions. Set goals related to the frequency and duration of your chair yoga practice, such as practicing three times per week for 30 minutes each session.

13. Set Mindfulness Goals: In addition to physical goals, consider setting goals related to mindfulness and stress reduction. Chair yoga offers an opportunity to cultivate mindfulness through breath awareness, meditation, and relaxation techniques. Set goals to incorporate these aspects into your practice to promote mental well-being alongside physical health.

14. Include Social and Community Goals: Chair yoga classes often provide a supportive and social environment, which can be beneficial for seniors. Consider setting goals related to building connections with others in your yoga class or participating in community events related to yoga or wellness. These social interactions can enhance motivation and enjoyment of your practice.

15. Adapt Goals as Needed: Be prepared to adapt your goals based on changes in your health, abilities, or personal circumstances. As you progress in your chair yoga practice, you may discover new goals or need to adjust existing ones to better align with your current needs and capabilities.

16. Celebrate Progress, Not Perfection: Focus on progress rather than perfection when working towards your goals. Celebrate small victories along the way, such as improvements in flexibility, increased energy levels, or better stress management. Acknowledge and appreciate the effort you put into your practice, regardless of the outcome.

17. Seek Professional Guidance: Consider seeking guidance from a certified yoga instructor or fitness professional who has experience working with seniors. They can help you set realistic goals based on your individual needs, provide personalized modifications, and offer encouragement and support throughout your journey.

18. Incorporate Lifestyle Goals: Chair yoga can complement other aspects of a healthy lifestyle, such as nutrition, hydration, and sleep. Consider setting goals related to these areas, such as incorporating more fruits and vegetables into your diet, staying hydrated throughout the day, or improving your sleep quality.

19. Stay Motivated with Variety: Keep your chair yoga practice engaging and enjoyable by incorporating variety into your routine. Set goals to explore different styles of chair yoga, try new poses or sequences, or attend workshops or retreats to deepen your practice and maintain motivation.

20. Practice Self-Compassion: Be kind to yourself throughout your journey. Accept that progress may be gradual, and setbacks are a natural part of the process. Practice self-compassion by treating yourself with patience, understanding, and self-care as you work towards your goals.

Staying Consistent with Chair Yoga Practice

Staying consistent with chair yoga practice as a senior requires dedication, motivation, and a few strategies to maintain regularity. Here's how you can stay consistent:

1. Establish a Routine: Set aside specific times each day or week for your chair yoga practice. Treat it like any other appointment or commitment and prioritize it in your schedule. Consistency is easier to maintain when yoga becomes a regular part of your daily or weekly routine.

2. Start Small: If you're new to chair yoga or have limited mobility, begin with shorter practice sessions and gradually increase the duration as you become more comfortable. Even just a few minutes of chair yoga each day can make a difference. Starting small makes it easier to stay consistent.

3. Find a Suitable Environment: Create a comfortable and inviting space for your chair yoga practice. Choose a quiet area with minimal distractions where you can focus on your practice without interruptions. Keep your yoga props, such as a chair, cushions, and any other accessories, easily accessible.

4. Set Realistic Goal : Establish achievable goals for your chair yoga practice, taking into account your current fitness level and any physical limitations. Setting realistic goals helps maintain motivation and allows you to track your progress over time.

5. Mix It Up: Keep your chair yoga practice interesting and engaging by varying your routine. Incorporate different poses, sequences, breathing techniques, and relaxation exercises to prevent boredom and maintain interest. Trying new things can help you stay motivated and committed to your practice.

6. Use Reminders: Set reminders or alarms on your phone, calendar, or other devices to prompt you to practice chair yoga. Having a visual or auditory cue can help ensure you don't forget your practice sessions, especially if you're busy or have a lot on your mind.

7. Practice Mindfulness: Cultivate mindfulness during your chair yoga practice by being fully present in the moment. Focus on the sensations of your breath, the movements of your body, and the feelings of relaxation and calmness. Mindfulness can enhance your enjoyment of yoga and motivate you to practice regularly.

8. Find Accountability: Share your chair yoga practice goals with a friend, family member, or caregiver who can offer support and encouragement. You can also join a chair yoga class or online community where you can connect with others who share similar goals and experiences.

9. Listen to Your Body: Be mindful of your body's needs and limitations during your chair yoga practice. If you're feeling tired or experiencing discomfort, modify poses or take a break as needed. Honoring your body's signals helps prevent injury and fosters a sustainable yoga practice.

10. Celebrate Your Progress: Acknowledge and celebrate your achievements and progress in your chair yoga practice, no matter how small. Recognize the effort and dedication you put into your practice, and use positive reinforcement to stay motivated and committed to consistent practice.

Certainly! Let's explore additional strategies to help you stay consistent with your chair yoga practice as a senior:

11. Adapt to Your Schedule: Recognize that life can be unpredictable, especially as a senior with various commitments and responsibilities. Be flexible and adaptable with your practice schedule. If you miss a planned session, don't be too hard on yourself. Instead, find alternative times or ways to fit in your practice, even if it means shorter sessions or practicing at a different time of day.

12. Create a Supportive Environment: Surround yourself with positive influences that encourage and support your chair yoga practice. Share your goals with supportive friends, family members, or caregivers who can provide encouragement and accountability. Consider joining a local chair yoga class or online community where you can connect with like-minded individuals and share experiences.

13. Set Up Visual Reminders: Place visual reminders of your chair yoga practice in prominent places where you'll see them regularly. This could be a sticky note on your bathroom mirror, a yoga mat unrolled in a designated corner of your living room, or a motivational quote related to yoga displayed in your home. These reminders serve as gentle prompts to prioritize and engage in your practice.

14. Keep It Simple and Accessible: Simplify your chair yoga practice to make it more accessible and manageable. Choose a few key poses and sequences that you enjoy and feel comfortable with, and focus on practicing them consistently. Keep your yoga props and accessories organized and easily accessible, so you can effortlessly transition into your practice whenever the opportunity arises.

15. Incorporate Mindful Movement Throughout the Day: Integrate mindful movement and stretching into your daily routine beyond dedicated chair yoga sessions. Take short breaks throughout the day to stretch and move your body gently. This could include simple seated stretches, shoulder rolls, neck rotations, or deep breathing exercises. These micro-practices help keep your body limber and promote overall well-being between formal yoga sessions.

16. Track Your Progress: Keep track of your chair yoga practice and progress using a journal, calendar, or digital app. Record the dates and durations of your practice sessions, along with any observations or reflections. Tracking your progress provides valuable feedback, helps you stay accountable, and allows you to celebrate milestones along the way.

17. Stay Inspired and Educated: Stay inspired and motivated by continuing to learn about chair yoga and its benefits. Explore books, articles, videos, and online resources related to chair yoga practice, mindfulness, and healthy aging. Attend workshops, seminars, or webinars led by experienced yoga instructors or wellness experts to deepen your knowledge and inspire your practice.

18. Practice Self-Compassion: Be compassionate with yourself on your yoga journey. Recognize that consistency is a process, and it's normal to experience ups and downs along the way. Be patient and kind to yourself, especially if you encounter challenges or setbacks. Approach your practice with a mindset of self-compassion, resilience, and determination.

<u>Conclusion</u>

<u>Recap of Key Points</u>

Here's a recap of the key points for chair yoga for weight loss for seniors over 60:

1. Benefits of Chair Yoga: Chair yoga offers numerous benefits for seniors over 60, including improved flexibility, strength, balance, and mental well-being. It can also aid in weight loss by promoting gentle movement, reducing stress, and enhancing mindfulness.

2. Physical Limitations: Seniors should be mindful of their physical limitations and adapt chair yoga poses accordingly. Modifications, props, and gradual progression are essential to ensure a safe and effective practice.

3. Setting Realistic Goals: Seniors should set realistic goals for their chair yoga practice, focusing on specific objectives such as improving flexibility, increasing muscle strength, or reducing stress levels. Using the SMART criteria (Specific, Measurable, Achievable, Relevant, Time-bound) can help in goal setting.

4. Staying Consistent: Consistency is key to seeing results from chair yoga for weight loss. Seniors can stay consistent by establishing a routine, starting small, finding a suitable environment, setting realistic goals, using reminders, and practicing mindfulness.

5. Adaptability and Flexibility: Seniors should be adaptable and flexible with their chair yoga practice, adjusting their schedule, environment, and goals as needed to accommodate changes in health, lifestyle, or circumstances.

6. Social Support and Accountability: Seeking social support and accountability from friends, family, caregivers, or fellow yoga practitioners can enhance motivation and consistency in chair yoga practice.

7. Self-Compassion and Celebration: Seniors should practice self-compassion and celebrate their progress, no matter how small. Acknowledging achievements and milestones along the way fosters a positive mindset and encourages continued effort.

8. Holistic Approach: Chair yoga for weight loss should be approached holistically, considering not only physical goals but also mental, emotional, and social well-being. Incorporating mindfulness, stress reduction techniques, social interaction, and lifestyle factors can contribute to overall success.

Final Words of Encouragement

Dear Senior Yogi,

As you embark on your chair yoga journey for weight loss, I want to offer you a final word of encouragement. Remember, this is a journey of self-discovery, self-care, and self-love.

Embrace each moment on the mat as an opportunity to connect with your body, mind, and spirit. Listen to your body's wisdom and honor its unique needs and limitations. Every breath, every movement is a step towards greater vitality and well-being.

Be patient with yourself. Progress may be gradual, but every small step forward is a triumph worth celebrating. Embrace the process, and trust in your ability to grow stronger, more flexible, and more resilient with each practice.

Stay consistent, even on days when motivation wanes. Your commitment to showing up for yourself, even in the face of challenges, is a testament to your strength and dedication.

Find joy in the journey. Cherish the moments of stillness and the moments of movement. Cultivate gratitude for the incredible gift of being able to nurture your body and soul through the practice of chair yoga.

Above all, be kind to yourself. You are embarking on a path of self-care and self-discovery that is both empowering and transformative. Trust in your inner wisdom, and know that you are capable of achieving your goals, one mindful breath at a time.

With love and encouragement,

Your Chair Yoga Companion